Collaborating for Health

Health care is increasingly under pressure. Budget crises are making collaboration and smart thinking essential, while increasing numbers of people with multiple long-term conditions make specialist models of health care increasingly inefficient – patients too often go from one specialist to another, duplicating effort and paying too little attention to the bigger picture of their health.

Collaborating for Health outlines a solution: community-oriented integrated care and health promotion. Designed to prevent the problems of fragmented care, this approach focuses on building teams, networks and communities for health and care at local level, where it is easier to see the range of factors that affect people's health. With the emphasis on partnership-working between primary care, public health and others, it allows clusters of general practices to share the work of integrating efforts for care and health improvement, and for non-medical organisations to lead parallel initiatives for health and care. Introducing both horizontal and vertical integration, Thomas presents ways to develop community-oriented integrated care in a sustainable way, and how to practise the skills in small ways before you have to perform on a big stage.

This guide is for anyone interested in how multidisciplinary primary care teams can orchestrate most aspects of health and care at local level, with timely specialist input.

Paul Thomas is a general practitioner in west London, professor of primary care research, education and development at the University of West London, UK, and honorary senior lecturer at Imperial College, UK. He is editor-in-chief of the *London Journal of Primary Care*, an international, Pubmed-cited journal that publishes case studies of integrated working in primary care and local communities.

Collaborating for Health

Paul Thomas

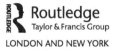

Routledge
Taylor & Francis Group

LONDON AND NEW YORK

First published 2018
by Routledge
2 Park Square, Milton Park, Abingdon, Oxon OX14 4RN

and by Routledge
711 Third Avenue, New York, NY 10017

Routledge is an imprint of the Taylor & Francis Group, an informa business

British Library Cataloguing-in-Publication Data
A catalogue record for this book is available from the British Library

Library of Congress Cataloging-in-Publication Data
Names: Thomas, Paul, 1955 January 20- author.
Title: Collaborating for health / Paul Thomas.
Description: Abingdon, Oxon ; New York, NY : Routledge, 2018. |
Includes bibliographical references and index.
Identifiers: LCCN 2017030665| ISBN 9781138300019 (hbk) |
ISBN 9781138300026 (pbk) | ISBN 9781315083711 (ebk)
Subjects: | MESH: Community Networks | Cooperative Behavior |
Delivery of Health Care, Integrated | Primary Health Care | Health
Promotion | United Kingdom
Classification: LCC RA427.8 | NLM WA 546 FA1 | DDC 362.1—dc23
LC record available at https://lccn.loc.gov/2017030665

ISBN: 978-1-138-30001-9 (hbk)
ISBN: 978-1-138-30002-6 (pbk)
ISBN: 978-1-315-08371-1 (ebk)

Typeset in Sabon
by Keystroke, Neville Lodge, Tettenhall, Wolverhampton

For Eunice my wife, David and Peter my sons, and Wendy my mother

Primary care

Public health

Guide

Practical   Integrated care

Collaborating for Health

Theories   Care pathways

Local health communities   Schools

Sustainable   Holistic

Models   Common sense

Citizenship   Co-evolving

Third way

Collaborating for health

Contents

About the author

Paul Thomas is a general practitioner in west London, professor of primary care research, education and development at University of West London and honorary senior lecturer at Imperial College. He is editor-in-chief of *London Journal of Primary Care*, which publishes case studies of integrated working in primary care and community contexts.

In 1989 he set up the Liverpool Primary Care Facilitation Project that used a community development approach to unite people in a broad coalition for health, hand in glove with the Liverpool Healthy City 2000 Project. Local multidisciplinary facilitation teams supported team-working in geographic areas of 70,000, supported by a university leadership course that helped them to become a pan-city network of leadership for collaborative practice. This project challenged orthodox ideas about how to go about sustainable change in health care, posing questions he puzzled over in his later work. He published theories and models that help to think about these questions in his 2006 book *Integrating Primary Health Care: leading, managing, facilitating* (Radcliffe Publishing)

He has seen challenges to managing practical and conceptual boundaries in health-care systems in different parts of the world – patient and practitioner boundaries in a Russian polyclinic, private and public boundaries in transplant surgery in India, medical and complementary therapy boundaries in a Chinese hospital, public health and primary care boundaries in Australia, insurance company boundaries in an American primary care clinic for the under-served, personal and village sanitation boundaries in rural Peru.

He has had many opportunities to see primary care innovations throughout the UK and debate theoretical and practical issues with people of experience. He was secretary of the Association of General Practices in Urban Deprived Areas (1990–95), Member of the King's Fund Urban Primary Care Network (1994–95), Chair of the National Advisory Committee for the National Primary Care Facilitation Programme (1998–2001), Member (then Deputy Chair) RCGP Inner City Task Force (1997–2001), Deputy Chair RCGP Health Inequalities Standing Group (2001–06) and Chair of the North-West London Faculty of the RCGP (2002–07).

In 1996, as senior lecturer at Imperial College, he set up the West London Research Network (WeLReN), which developed multi-perspective participatory research in primary care. At Thames Valley University (now University of West London) he developed leadership courses for primary care groups (2001–08). As Clinical Director at Ealing Primary Care Trust (2007–11) and Clinical Lead for Ealing Clinical

Commissioning Group (2011–13), he developed the Southall Initiative for Integrated Care, applying what he had learned about integrated working to clusters of practices and systems of care.

He is presently exploring low-cost, systematic ways for primary care, public health and out-of-hours practitioners to develop *local health communities* in west London.

Acknowledgements

I remember the people of Liverpool with great affection. Between 1989 and 1995 we created a grand alliance for health and care. I still owe thanks to those who collaborated to show that the principles of comprehensive primary health care can be systematically translated into practice – the Primary Care Facilitation Project, Medical Audit Advisory Group, Healthy City 2000 Project, Public Health, City Council, Local Medical Committee, Liverpool Occupational Health Project, Trade Unions, Health Authority and Family Health Services Authority. We all witnessed the profound and long-term effects of our collective actions, like ripples in all directions when a single boat crosses an empty harbour.

These days harbours are criss-crossed by ever more boats travelling in every direction. It's almost impossible to see the effect of any one intervention, let alone a strategic set. This led me to question the value of both top-down and bottom-up approaches to change, and pilot ways to link different kinds of innovation from different parts of the system. I learned that small interventions can have value of their own and also be positioned to enhance others, if we pay attention to the linkages. So I owe thanks to people in London who supported projects to pilot such linkage.

I want to thank my many friends in West London Research Network (WeLReN), University of West London, Imperial College, Ealing Primary Care Trust and Clinical Commissioning Group, Ealing Mental Health and Wellbeing Service, Southall general practices, Cuckoo Lane Surgery, Central Ealing Health Network, Royal College of General Practitioners London Faculties, London Journal of Primary Care, and London Central and West Unscheduled Care Service. With full support of senior people in these organisations we were able to pilot *development and research practices* that supported geographically based *local health communities*, whose boundaries were aligned with hospital outreach *'tier two' clinics for long-term conditions*. We piloted an *applied research unit* that developed shared leadership teams to facilitate learning and change across multiple disciplinary boundaries. We set up *a web-based journal* to publish *case studies of integrated care* and facilitate *international discussion* of the emerging discussions.

I have again been struck by how unused most practitioners and managers are to systems-thinking and participatory processes to organisational learning and change, and indeed how threatening they are to some. My experience is that the approach always works, but it is always difficult – perhaps because it challenges linear ways of thinking and vested interests.

The experience that best showed to me how primary care can galvanise local contributions to health and care was in Soweto, South Africa in 1994 and again in 1997. Here the nurse practitioners were the GPs, supported by a medical GP (Andrew Truscott) and specialists when needed. These same nurse practitioners were also leaders in the local churches, as 'bare-foot' public health promoters and community developers. The poverty and inequalities so manifest there, coupled with a newfound sense of hope, made it clear that comprehensive integration is possible. But it needs long-term infrastructure and vision. It needs local multidisciplinary leadership teams that unite people across boundaries by facilitating group learning, emphasising positive things and using crises as a force for good. Really difficult situations can indeed be the best seed-beds of comprehensive cooperation.

I have learned that the natural process of successful change is two steps forward, then three steps back, then (sometimes) something happens to galvanise people and everyone starts to work together (not always by any means) to co-create ten steps forward. I have learned that it requires humour and patience – and trusted friends.

Special thanks goes to some individuals who were always there. I could always rely on them for friendship, sound advice and thoughtful critique. Whenever I am stuck, I ask myself what advice they would give me, and just this thought often helps me to become unstuck, or at least recognise that I am in a no-win situation. Thanks to Janet Hayes, John Horder, David Colin Thome, Siobhan Clarke, Baljeet Ruprah-Shah, Ricky Banarsee, Paul Quin, Peter Cawley, Maurice Keane, John Launer, Ray Ison, Will Miller, Vicki Doyle, Lynne Madden, Peter Sainsbury, John Macdonald, Sam Everington, Ewan Ferlie, Mark Spencer, David Morris, Chris Brophy, Raj Chandok, Neha Unadkat, Peter Kinch and Kurt Stange. I was greatly helped in the drafting of this book by the wise advice of Peter and Kurt.

Also thanks to the many friends, both parents and teachers, in my sons' schools – Malorees School and Cardinal Vaughan Memorial School. The striking similarity of the challenges in health care and schools have been the subject of many helpful discussions, fuelled of course by countless cups of tea.

Forewords

Professor Mayur Lakhani, CBE; RCGP President and GP;
Chair of West Leicestershire Clinical Commissioning Group;
past Chair of the Royal College of GPs; Chairman of The
National Council for Palliative Care

This is a powerful book and an important contribution to the literature on integrated care. Its timing is impeccable, coming as it does with the publication of the NHS Sustainability and Transformation Plans (STPs), which are aimed at creating accountable care systems for integrated care and in which system leadership is critical – the raison d'être for this book in my view.

As someone closely involved in STPs, I have found this book immensely helpful. It is essential reading for anyone involved in STPs, particularly in creating primary and community integrated care services at scale. As a minimum, Thomas's three-tier model of long-term conditions management is a winner and should be adopted widely and quickly to improve outcomes and deliver better value.

The book not only provides the evidence base for change but also practical support with, for example 'live manuals' and comprehensive skills checklists. I like the suggestions of 'seasons of learning and change' and his model of connectedness (as the link, glue and cell) is memorable. To cap it all the book is littered with enjoyable references to the arts and literature with quotes from Shakespeare, Kipling and others.

Lord Ara Darzi, Director of the Institute of Global Health
Innovation, Imperial College London

Whilst fulfilling my role as health minister, I produced the *High Quality Care for All* report in 2008, within which I highlighted that 'for the NHS to be sustainable in the 21st century it needs to focus on improving health as well as treating sickness'. In order for this to be achieved there is an urgent need to find practical ways to integrate community-based efforts of personal care and population health, and combine this with the efforts of specialists and generalists. This insightful book offers a sustainable and evidenced way to action this whilst delving into the difficulties that we face both practically and theoretically implementing such strategies.

As the health-care system faces increased burden from ageing populations and rising rates of chronic disease, the system needs to adapt to ensure that we tackle the inefficiencies of fragmented care and improve the integration of all services. This brilliantly perceptive and motivational book inspires everyone from scientists, health-care professionals, social workers, patients, families and policymakers to engage with their communities and take a lead in integrating approaches to care and health. It clearly demonstrates how the use of behavioural insights can maximise the impact of the most effective heath-care promotion strategies. It provides examples of successful extended primary care teams and encourages readers to develop their own case study, using a proven framework. *Collaborating for Health* will undoubtedly inspire its readers to take charge of their community in order to improve the health outcomes and quality of life of those around them.

Dr Victoria Tzortziou-Brown, NHS Tower Hamlets CCG Lead on Integrated Care and Research; RCGP London Chair and Joint Honorary Secretary RCGP

Health care worldwide is recognised as a complex, adaptive system with often a complicated design and a non-linear, ambiguous, dynamic and unpredictable nature. A common approach to dealing with complexity is to reduce or constrain it by dividing the system into smaller, separate parts. However, such an approach is not always appropriate for a system whose behaviour cannot be expressed as simply a sum of the behaviour of its interconnected parts. This is increasingly being recognised and it explains the drive towards more collaboration and integration across and between health and care organisations.

Probably the most important aspect of such integration is the cultural change required to be able to challenge and overcome behavioural barriers and work towards a common vision whilst learning with and from each other. Health-care professionals and policymakers need to develop foresight and insight, to accept the complexity within health-care organisations and recognise the importance of promoting a learning system and supporting creative and distributed leadership at all levels.

Future leaders need to understand complexity and acquire the expertise to operate and evolve within a complex environment in order to be able to foster resilient and adaptable health-care systems. This book summarises beautifully the interconnected, emergent nature of health organisations and offers practical wisdom on how to develop the necessary skills to effect positive and meaningful change within them. It guides readers to find their own answers within their health communities. The author's profundity and insight into collaborative, system learning will appeal not just to front-line health-care professionals but also educators, commissioners, researchers and policymakers, and will hopefully inspire many to take positive action. After all, as the book says, 'community-oriented integrated care needs everyone to contribute to connected communities for health'.

Professor Lynne Madden, Associate Dean at The University of Notre Dame Australia; President of the Australasian Faculty of Public Health Medicine, Royal Australasian College of Physicians

Fragmented health care is not much fun for anyone; it is confusing, frightening and exhausting for patients and their carers, frustrating for insightful practitioners, wasteful for the system, unsafe and leads to poorer health outcomes. Consequently health systems are exploring more patient-centred approaches, seeking to achieve the Alma Alta goal of comprehensive primary health care, which, as Paul highlights, is the Holy Grail for helping people to have healthier and happier lives. Around the world health systems are trying different approaches to locality-based, patient-centred, integrated care, focused on improving people's lives. Many look to the UK for examples of practice; the honest acknowledge that transformational change is hard to do and a long-term strategy.

As Paul points out, the goal of integrated care means different things in different places; places are also moving at different paces. While often the focus is improving the quality of care for people who are frail or elderly or have multiple morbidities this guide argues for a broad focus for community-orientated integrated care of 'health' rather than only 'disease'. This guide contains resources that will help no matter what the state and stage of development. Indeed, it is a resource applicable to any person or organisation seeking to engage in collaborative activity and/or change.

By adopting a 'learning by doing' approach it encourages reflective practitioners to build their own capacity for teamwork, integrated care and engagement with complexity. However, it should not be left to individuals acting alone to define and build their competencies. Organisations responsible for the education of health-care professionals – universities, professional colleges, associations and workplaces – should consider the essential competencies for evolving practice. We all bear responsibility for the capacity of people to engage successfully with these processes.

Paul has been driven throughout his professional career by the belief that you can change things for the better. This guide is the result of his 30-plus years of working within primary care and across sectors to strengthen the health system's capacity to delivery better health outcomes for people and communities. Throughout, Paul has valued public health's capacity to help join the dots to make the system more effective for individuals and populations and achieve 'Health for All'.

He encourages us to retain the faith that committed people aligned can make a big difference. Dipping in and out of this manual will give you lots of different perspectives on how you might nudge a system along a pathway by strengthening democratic processes and engaging with people and communities. The manual is full of ways to help create change processes for organisations but also at a personal level. I commend it to you.

Professor Kurt Stange, Case Western Reserve University, USA, and family physician; editor of *Annals of Family Medicine*

This is a wise and practical book. It is about achieving quality health care on the ground while keeping the big picture of personal and population health, equity and sustainability in mind and in action.

This kind of thinking, and the actions it leads to, are particularly needed around the world at this moment because the disutility of fragmented, reductionist approaches to improvement is apparent, but the alternative isn't. This book makes it clear how an integrated approach to health care and health promotion can be accomplished by new ways of understanding and acting – teamwork that develops relationships, systems-thinking and cycles of learning and change at the local level that can solve some of the most apparently intractable problems of individuals, communities and the whole population.

The book's wisdom comes from the experience of an author who has devoted his life to helping diverse individuals and groups work together towards a common goal of healthier people and communities. Paul Thomas's deep personal experience and pragmatic knowledge is complemented by his search for the transportable principles that underlie collaborative learning and coordinated change. These principles reflect systems science in action. These radical yet straightforward concepts move health care and health promotion from delivery of commodities to development of healing and health promoting relationships. We need this approach to reduce wasteful expenditure, to overcome depersonalising fragmentation and to advance healthy populations.

The book's practicality stems from its 'how to' approach. Bring your own case study – the current wicked problem that you find so vexing that it seems like there is nowhere to start. The book will walk you through how to get your head around its complexities at whatever scale matters to you – from the individual to the organisation to the community and the system. It will help you to begin systematic action towards sustainable change. In addition to immediately actionable steps, the book contains surprising and satisfying bites of practical wisdom, and useful references that provide deeper background for each section. Whether you are a practitioner, a change agent, a policymaker – the ideas, experience and hope in these pages will help you fruitfully move between action and reflection to develop healing, health promoting relationships.

These pages reveal an authentic way to come to grips with the challenges of working in complex systems. They show how to build and sustain trusted human relationships that bind people together with passion as well as contracts. The hands-on tools and useful theories presented here provide a compelling alternative to the mechanistic mental models usually used to describe integration. They make integrated working feel human and rich — about health as well as disease, about solutions as well as problems.

Read the very useful Introduction and decide where to start. Then dive in.

Endorsements

Professor Ewan Ferlie, King's College London, UK

This is an interesting, important and relevant book that will be a valuable resource for all leaders and change agents in trying to change, improve and integrate primary care services and to so in a system-based way. It obviously addresses a key health-policy agenda. The text combines expositions of useful organisational concepts, mini-cases, practical exercises, references to further sources and visualisations in an attractive and accessible mix. It should be a key reference point for all those seeking to promote community-orientated and more integrated primary care.

Professor Peter Whitehouse, Case Western Reserve University, USA, and University of Toronto, Canada; Strategic Advisor in Innovation Baycrest Health Center; President, Intergenerational Schools International

This book and its author, Paul Thomas, are conceptual, practical and wise guides to the health-care organisational change we all want. Using stories that make sense and ideas that challenge we are led on both revolutionary flights of inspiring imagination and into grounded lived experiences. The book convinces us that healthy systems are possible and necessary in these challenging times. Paul himself, his journal and inspiring colleagues have been guides for me as I struggle to integrate primary care and public health in community settings. The book is inter-generative as we reach between disciplines and professions to go beyond to a better more healthy future.

Siobhan Clarke, Managing Director of Your Healthcare CIC

If you are looking for a definitive text that will afford both the supporting theory and the practical tools to make brilliant care happen for brilliant people then this is it. People live in communities; they thrive in communities and yet when we talk about health and social care systems we tend to make only paltry reference to the most critical of operating systems – the social economy of families and neighbourhood. Within these neighbourhoods, co-existing alongside people in their homes, are our primary care colleagues. Has there ever been a better time to utilise and build on the strength and the continuity of relationships that primary care offers? Make great of use of this book and draw on the wisdom that it reminds us that we hold. Let us organise our worlds differently and collaborate generously for better health for everyone.

Professor David Colin-Thomé, Manchester Business School, UK, and GP; former National Clinical Director for Primary Care; Medical Adviser for Commissioning and System Reform

If like me, you are frustrated that R&D usually focuses solely on research and you wish to focus on development – this book is for you (although in the spirit of this book they should be as one).

If you value trusted relationships in shared care and collaborative health promotion at local, community level – this book is for you.

If you wish to be guided by an experienced, highly intelligent and intellectual general medical practitioner who is an expert in facilitation and community development and yet in my personal knowledge of him does not 'lose the common touch' – this author is for you.

Professor Sir Sam Everington, OBE; GP and Barrister

The NHS is facing a massive challenge with increased demand, an ageing population and advances in science and technology. Primary care has always been the jewel in the crown of the NHS and its expansion and development is seen now by government and policymakers as the way to resolve the challenge. Analysis shows it needs to expand its offering by a third as described in the NHS England 'Five Year Forward View'.

We need to shift care into the community and support patients to manage their health and wellbeing. Social prescribing in general practice will be one of the key projects along with integrated care. Why is this important for patients? Just one example relates to end-of-life care, where typically 60 per cent of patients die in hospital and yet nearly all would prefer to die at home surrounded by their loved ones. Supporting patients at home would be a far more compassionate service for patients, deliver great primary care and deliver much better value for money.

This book shows us how we can deliver this change with practical examples. It is essential reading for anyone passionate about primary care and the NHS.

Professor Rebecca Malby, London South Bank University, UK

In the Western world the traditional model of primary care is broken. The foundations for our health services, of demand being curtailed by cure was false. Communities and services need to forge new relationships that are more about 'co' than about expert and recipient, to support people to better health and to better use our health-service resources. Bringing the talent, insight and research of health-service professionals together with the assets of communities in a collaboration will take a real focus on relationships, and on being adaptable together. This book charts the complex change required from the list-based GP to a population-based health model. It provides a wealth of tools for inquiry and change that support the transition. Start anywhere in the book and go everywhere.

Paul Stubbings, Headmaster of Cardinal Vaughan Memorial School, UK

I was struck when I started this innovative book by how much it was applicable to my field – education. It quickly became clear, though, that this is precisely the point that is so lucidly made: it is very apparent that we are all part of the same unfurling narrative. This study shows that it is not so much that it's all about inter-connectivity – there is actually nothing but inter-connectivity. This has important implications for how we set about devising and delivering the school curriculum.

Professor Raj Chandok, Buckinghamshire New University, UK, and GP; Vice Chair, NHS Ealing Clinical Commissioning Group

Paul is and has always been a passionate advocate for innovation and quality improvement in primary care. He has also been a great friend to me and many newly qualified GPs and challenged them to develop fulfilling and successful careers, always guiding and helping by supportive timely advice.

A decade and a half ago he was articulating coherently his vision of health care (primary, community and secondary), mental health care and social care professionals working closely and focusing on the delivery of care on populations of 50,000 patients; he referred to this as 'local health communities'. The aspiration was for an integrated patient-centred care model with a clear focus on improved communication and teamworking. This was a very avant garde concept at the time but is now the basis on the NAPC Primary Care Home model and the multi-speciality care provider model described in the NHS Five Year Forward View. The fact that the local health community vision is therefore now being realised is a testament to Paul's radical ideas being understood and implemented many years later.

Catherine Millington-Sanders, RCGP/Marie Curie National Clinical End of Life Care Champion

Thought-provoking! An enjoyable read for professionals through to commissioners and policymakers. Thomas's book is a major contribution to health care and inspires transformational change, especially for care for people with advanced serious illness and end-of-life needs. Perfect for GPs and clinicians in primary care, the book provides insight and practical advice on a community-oriented integrated care approach. Using interesting case studies, evidence and reflection exercises throughout, it manages to bring to life strategies and drivers, not merely for the treatment of diseases but to enable local society collaboration for whole population health. Thomas illuminates how dynamic inquiry can be used to enable real-time strategic change. Crucially, the book engages how learning communities can embrace openness in order for learning and change to be the cultural norm. Leaders will not regret experiencing their own adventure when reading his methods to balance their own inner peace when confidence or control of their vision is threatened! In summary, a glorious banquet to feast your eyes and open your minds.

Who is the book for?

This book is for anyone who wants to know how to engage large numbers of people in collaborative activities for a healthy society – schools, faith groups and voluntary groups, for example. In particular it focuses on how primary care, in partnership with public health and others, can coordinate health and care at local levels, and in so doing advance the World Health Organization vision of comprehensive primary health care – health and care are responsibilities of all citizens and all sectors of society.

It advocates a *learning organisation* approach – parallel cycles of collaborative learning and coordinated change interconnect to create *learning communities*, building relationships and stimulating innovation throughout whole systems. Control is maintained by holding each other to negotiated agreements. It requires a multi-perspective, 'both–and' approach to most things. It means responsibilities as well as rights, self-care as well as care from and for others. It requires multi-method evaluation, complex interventions, systems thinking, multidisciplinary shared leadership and a dynamic, co-adapting understanding of reality.

Each part targets a different kind of reader, so revisits the same ideas in different ways:

- Part I – policymakers
- Part II – leaders of community-based organisations
- Part III – leaders of collaborative working in geographic areas
- Part IV – students of the science of integrated working in health care
- Part V – students of organisational development in health care

The models described in the book help people from different backgrounds to work well with others, across ideological and organisational boundaries. They are what Charles Handy calls 'Empty Raincoat' models like *care plans* and *live manuals* – they may look solid from the outside, but you fill them with what makes sense in your specific situation. They have been tested in the UK with primary care practitioners (e.g. GPs) and community care practitioners (e.g. community nurses, mental health and allied health professionals, social workers) and the organisations that relate to them – hospitals, trusts, clinical commissioning groups, public health, local authorities, universities, schools and voluntary groups.

The models inter-link, potentially applied at scale to nurture comprehensive collaboration throughout health care, and even throughout society, helping to counter-balance the inward-looking instincts of modern citizens. The book also describes the skills that people need to interact creatively with others to build trusted relationships. These skills can be learned at every stage of life. The book explains why multi-level co-evolution matters, and why networks of boundary-spanning leadership teams help to bring it about.

Health-care policymakers in many countries may find the principles and models relevant. You don't have to use them all – start where you can and do more when you can. Throughout the world the winds are blowing in the direction of comprehensive primary health care. Budget crises make collaboration and smart thinking essential. Increasing numbers of people with multiple long-term conditions make specialist models of health care increasingly inefficient – patients too often go from one specialist to another, duplicating effort and paying too little attention to the bigger picture of their health.

The book has something to offer other readers. Everyone in society needs to contribute to environments for health. The processes outlined here describe a form of participatory democracy that politicians may find interesting. It presents a way to think about the inter-dependence of individuals and communities, and different dimensions of health – spiritual, physical, mental and social. In many ways this is old wisdom – things that have been known for thousands of years, applied to a modern context.

Bring your own case study

Real examples bring dry theory to life, so you will benefit by bringing your own case study to the chapters – perhaps something you are trying to change in a borough, general practice or a network of practices. Your case could be something quite different – a school, your own family or community, for example. However modest it is, use it. The 'real world' is messy and unpredictable and any one theory is rarely adequate. A case study helps to remember this and see why a participatory, organic, learning approach helps.

Describing your case study

Chapter 11 describes case study research. To describe your 'case study' you do not have to be so rigorous. You simply need to describe a project that you are working on in a way that helps you to consider whether the exercises at the end of each chapter are useful to you or not.

A quick way to bring your case to mind is to speak it aloud – to a mirror, into a voice recorder or to a friend. Speaking it aloud can make it easier to hear what you want to say. Saying it to another offers them the opportunity to seek clarification about things that are unclear.

A simple way to structure your ideas is to use the same old format when advertising an event – Who? What? When? Where? Why?

Who: This case is called 'Integrating Primary Care in Test Site'.

What: Integrating Primary Care in Test Site is an initiative to integrate the working of ten general practices in a locality of 50,000 population with the work of public health and specialists from a local hospital. It involves four half-day workshops a year at which representatives of the disciplines devise modest projects that help them to align their ways of working. A multidisciplinary leadership team meets monthly to continue the work in between the workshops.

When: It began in 2014, building from pilot work that started in 2012.

Where: It operates in Test Site, an inner-city area of Test Town.

Why: The fragmented nature of local health care was causing costly duplication of effort and a sense of isolation of local practitioners. We thought that the combination of modest multidisciplinary projects with educational updating would help to build relationships between different disciplines and organisations, to mutual advantage.

When you have a case study in mind, ask yourself 'What do I want from integration?' Perhaps you want the whole system to be more coherent and more efficient? Be honest about your own self-interest as well as your aim(s) for the system. Perhaps you want to keep your job? To persuade the world of your way of seeing things? To hit your targets? To achieve personal goals? You don't have to abandon self-interest in favour of the interest of the system as a whole – but you must not confuse the two.

Try these exercises to improve your understanding of the dynamics within your case study and things you might do to chart a successful course.

1   **Brainstorm:** At the top of a large sheet of (flip chart) paper write the name of your case study and your aim(s) for its development. Brainstorm (list) things that are working well (these are things you can build from), things that are not working well (these are things you need to better understand) and the teams, individuals and organisations who are the actors who might be able to improve things. Colour-code the three categories (e.g. yellow, orange and purple).
2   **System diagram:** On a second sheet of paper indicate with small circles (e.g. in black) the main relevant organisations and teams and their lines of accountability.
3   **Populate the system diagram:** Using the same colour-code, indicate on the system diagram the location of things from your brainstorm – things going well, not well and the actors. Draw lines between them to show how they affect each other, using a fourth colour (e.g. red) to indicate direct power and a fifth (e.g. blue) for influence. Use arrow heads to show which ways the power flows. Use dotted and lines of different thickness to indicate strong and weak effects ('ties'). Indicate with a sixth colour (e.g. green) those you might be able to influence.
4   **Surface hidden factors:** On the system diagram, add in less obvious things that might impact on the system. These could be 'off-stage' individuals with formal or informal roles who influence others, or funding sources, staff sickness, cultural conflicts, lack of skill and so on.
5   **Reflect and plan:** Now stand back and look at your system map. Where might modest interventions have a big impact on integration, by harnessing existing forces? And particularly by working in the places that you can influence (coloured green). Would it help if any strong ties were weakened, or weak ones strengthened, or new ones created? Are new components needed? Try adding them and see how it feels. You may need to redraw the system diagram many times. Explain the diagram to a trusted friend who doesn't know the system and ask if it makes sense to them.
6   **See other perspectives:** Now put yourself in the shoes of different individuals on the diagram. Would they see the system as you see it? What are they likely to say if you ask them how to improve the system? What might be a winning approach with them?
7   **Plan a collaborative project:** What project is most likely to engage the actors you want to engage – improvement project, rapid appraisal, large group event, live manual?

The first 12 chapters invite you to add to your case study:

1   **Identify champions for change:** Identify individuals, groups and networks in your case study that are ready to take a fuller role in developing community-oriented

integrated care and health promotion. Consider ways to connect their activities with those of others in your case study. What projects might they lead?

2 **Create a care plan:** Sit down with someone (e.g. a patient or friend) and create a care plan for them. In what ways was this valuable?

3 **Identify relationship-building activities:** Identify existing events and activities that stimulate creative conversations between different actors. Consider ways that they could be connected for greater effect (e.g. by cascading ideas from one to another or a shared project).

4 **Engage strategic partners:** Consider organisational partner(s) in your case study who could help move forward your plans for development. Design a pilot project with them.

5 **Devise an annual cycle of activity:** Develop an annual timetable of activity. Use *participatory action research* to lead a pilot project(s). Consider what routinely gathered data could contribute to evaluation of the project(s).

6 **Write a live manual:** Consider which topics in your case study would most benefit from a live manual. Who will write it? Ask them to.

7 **Use techniques that see parts and wholes:** Use an organic image, theory or method that helps to see the connection between parts and wholes in your case study. Does it help you to see what is going on? Does it help you to see what to do?

8 **Assess your developmental needs:** Go through the Appendix: Skills to lead community-oriented integrated care. List the skills you want to develop within one year and five years. Note skills you want your teams to develop.

9 **Engage stakeholders:** Write a strategy to engage different constituents in the annual cycle of learning and change in your case study.

10 **Hold a whole system event:** Hold a whole system event led by a shared leadership team.

11 **Pilot research methods:** Use a range of research methods to illuminate aspects of your case study.

12 **Devise a personal plan for self-actualisation.**

Introduction

Comprehensive primary health care develops trusted partnerships

This book explores practical ways to achieve the holy grail of comprehensive primary health care – whole society collaboration for whole population health. In particular it explores how primary care, in partnership with public health, specialists and others, can facilitate activities that bring together – integrate – the efforts of people from different parts of the system.

It is about trusted partnerships. To integrate care people need to relate to each other in ways that work. Success combines three different kinds of relationship. Direct control and 'line management' are good for simple short-term actions. Contractual relationships allow people to know what to expect of each other. Mutually responsive relationships allow people to co-create new things. A 'trusted relationship' combines all three: we take direct, individual action when needed; we do what we said we would do when that is needed; we respond creatively to others when that is needed. You know when the balance is right because it works – it feels right and it makes things happen, in a good way.

Health-care workers need to improve overall health as well as treat diseases. There is little point in curing someone's illness if it fails to improve their health. Health means having a spring in your step and a smile on your face; it means feeling that your life story makes sense as a whole and your relationships are meaningful. Many factors other than medicine affect this. Success comes from synchronising the work of health-care practitioners with the work of many others, so the combined effect is more than the sum of the individual efforts.

This book explores how to enable multiple-way synchrony. Family medicine/general practice is well placed to contribute because its practioners regularly communicate with people from all parts of the system and we operate at local level – where people live out their lives. Here, it is easier to see the multiple factors that help or hinder the health of individuals, families and communities. Here, it is obvious why healthy environments are ones that support shared-care, self-care and healthy living. Here, it is obvious that all citizens need to contribute to a healthy society.

Awareness that all citizens need to contribute to healthy societies found international agreement at the 1978 World Health Organization (WHO) conference in Alma-Ata, then the capital of Kazakhstan in the former USSR. In total, 134 member states of the WHO and United Nations Children's Fund (UNICEF), and 67 international organisations concluded a set of ten shared values that underpin what they called *(comprehensive) primary health care.*

Primary health care (PHC) is much more than primary care. Declaration VII of the Alma Ata Declaration states:

> Primary health care . . . involves, in addition to the health sector, all related sectors and aspects of national and community development, in particular agriculture, animal husbandry, food, industry, education, housing, public works, communications and other sectors; and demands the coordinated efforts of those sectors.

Public health is charged with achieving PHC – a healthy society where citizens care about others, beyond their self-interests. However, PHC is not so easy to achieve. Different people think differently about how to treat diseases, how to improve health, and their roles in both. Many are unable to see beyond their own mindsets. The combative approach of curative medicine (e.g. killing bacteria with antibiotics) thinks differently from immunisation and acupuncture that help a body to help itself. Different traditions more or less emphasise physical health (e.g. exercise), social health (e.g. relationships), mental health (e.g. being able to think clearly) and spiritual health (e.g. feeling internally centred). Each has its own theories and language. Bringing them together in meaningful ways is not straightforward.

Different approaches to health improvement also need different approaches to evaluation. Direct effects, like that of an antibiotic, can be evaluated by a laboratory (*positivist*) approach. Complicated effects like social networks need a *critical theory* approach to see hidden connections. Building a learning organisation needs participation in the processes of inquiry and change, as is revealed in a *constructivist* approach. Multiple methods evaluation is needed to reveal both short- and long-term effects of complex interventions.

Different aspects of integration even require different understandings of 'integration'. Disease care requires 'hard', 'vertical integration' – care pathways that share care between generalists and specialists. Collaboration for a healthy society requires 'soft', 'horizontal integration' – a dynamic process of shared leadership between different disciplines.

Different understandings can cause a 'Tower of Babel' effect – incoherent noise. To reconcile multiple voices, we have to see things from many different perspectives, appreciate what others contribute and build from the positive rather than merely attack the negative. This requires deep listening – to what others say and also to what they mean to say but perhaps struggle to put into words. We must also listen to what we each ourselves say and mean, and surface the assumptions that lie behind our words. Then people need to develop a shared story – however divided may be their roots, integration means that they must painstakingly develop a story that has a positive, intertwined new heart.

The book presents methods that facilitate deep listening between people who think they have nothing in common; and ways to link various conversational strands over time. The methods allow people to repeatedly dip in and out each other's lives, over time, in ways that permit separate, individual journeys as well as intense moments of shared travel.

This book shows how overlapping cycles of learning and change can integrate multiple contributions to PHC. The first three parts contain models – Part I for policy, Part II for community-based organisations like general practices, Part III for local health communities. Parts IV and V explain more fully theories mentioned along the way. If you want to understand the history of integrated care and why general practice should have a strong role in leading it, read Chapters 13 and 14. If you want to understand health (rather than disease) and how to interact in healthy ways with others, read Chapters 15 and 18. If you want to know how to evaluate complex interventions, read Chapters 11 and 16.

Each model can be useful on its own, but a combination is much more powerful because they feed off each other. Linking them is not always possible, especially when this conflicts with local expectations, so start where you can and do more later. It also requires disciplined adherence to the 'rules of the road' – not everyone wants to drive on the designated side of the road. So expect the journey to be stuttering, and when things seem to go backwards, gravitate with good humour to where there is energy for a next stage.

The approach is based on cycles of collaborative learning and coordinated change. This is how individuals, organisations and systems learn and change. This *learning organisation* approach is quite different from traditional structural bureaucracy. You will need patience – people need at least three cycles before they see the power of the approach. The cycles work best when they sit alongside more traditional mechanisms of control, providing a way for 'bottom-up' and 'top-down' approaches to powerfully enrich each other.

Remember, the models are not prescriptive. They are connected opportunities for people to work together, and from this develop trusted relationships that provide the binding force of integration. You will need to use them in ways that make sense in your situation.

Comprehensive primary health care – more important than ever

Since 1978 the PHC vision has been pursued by countries throughout the world in one way or another. International policy has evolved. In 2000 8 *Millennium Development*

Goals were described and in 2015 these were revised into 17 *Sustainable Development Goals* with 169 targets covering a broad range of sustainable development issues.

In the early days, comprehensive PHC quickly gave way to targeted PHC – things like immunisation and breast feeding. In 2008, Margaret Chan, WHO Director-General, explained that the broader vision of PHC needs to be rediscovered because it is key to solving serious problems in contemporary societies.

 World Health Organization. *Primary Health Care – Now More than Ever.* www. who.int/whr/2008/

Chan's 2008 WHO Report described three such problems:

- The substantial progress in health over recent decades has been deeply unequal, often with health inequalities within countries.
- Ageing . . . increase the burden of chronic disorders. Many individuals present with complex symptoms and multiple illnesses [that] challenge service delivery to develop more integrated and comprehensive case management.
- System's failure requires a system's solution – not a temporary remedy . . . health systems seem to be drifting from one short-term priority to another, increasingly fragmented and without a clear sense of direction . . . left to their own devices, health systems do not gravitate naturally towards the goals of health for all through primary health care as articulated in the Declaration of Alma Ata.

The Report identifies three particularly worrisome trends:

- Health systems that focus disproportionately on a narrow offer of specialized curative care
- Health systems where a command and control approach to disease control, focused on short-term results, is fragmenting service delivery
- Health systems where a hands-off or laissez-faire approach to governance has allowed unregulated commercialization of health to flourish.

It has this to say about challenges for healthy public policy:

- Public policy-making is about more than classical public health. Primary care and social protection reforms critically depend on choosing health-systems policies, such as those related to essential drugs, technology, human resources and financing, which are supportive of the reforms that promote equity and people-centred care.
- They can no longer be content with mere administration of the system: they have to become learning organizations. This requires inclusive leadership that engages with a variety of stakeholders beyond the boundaries of the public sector, from clinicians to civil society, and from communities to researchers and academia.

It has this to say about how experience has shifted the focus of the PHC movement:

From	To
Extended access to a basic package of health interventions and essential drugs for the rural poor	Transformation and regulation of existing health systems, aiming for universal access and social health protection
Concentration on mother and child health	Dealing with the health of everyone in the community
Focus on a small number of selected diseases, primarily infectious and acute	A comprehensive response to people's expectations and needs, spanning the range of risks and illnesses
Improvement of hygiene, water, sanitation and health education at village level	Promotion of healthier lifestyles and mitigation of the health effects of social and environmental hazards
Simple technology for volunteer, non-professional community health workers	Teams of health workers facilitating access to and appropriate use of technology and medicines
Participation as the mobilization of local resources and health-centre management through local health committees	Institutionalized participation of civil society in policy dialogue and accountability mechanisms
Government-funded and delivered services with a centralized top-down management	Pluralistic health systems operating in a globalized context
Management of growing scarcity and downsizing	Guiding the growth of resources for health towards universal coverage
Management of growing scarcity and downsizing	Guiding the growth of resources for health towards universal coverage
Bilateral aid and technical assistance	Global solidarity and joint learning
Primary care as the antithesis of the hospital	Primary care as coordinator of a comprehensive response at all levels
PHC is cheap and requires only a modest investment	PHC is not cheap: it requires considerable investment, but it provides better value for money than its alternatives

The Report concludes with four sets of reforms that require 'delicate trade-offs and negotiation with multiple stakeholders':

1   **Universal coverage reforms** – that ensure that health systems contribute to health equity, social justice and the end of exclusion
2   **Service delivery reforms** – reforms that reorganize health services as primary care, i.e. around people's needs and expectations, so as to make them more socially relevant and more responsive to the changing world while producing better outcomes
3   **Public policy reforms** – reforms that secure healthier communities, by integrating public health actions with primary care and by pursuing healthy public policies across sectors

4   **Leadership reforms** – reforms that replace disproportionate reliance on command and control on one hand, and laissez-faire disengagement of the state on the other, by the inclusive, participatory, negotiation-based leadership required by the complexity of contemporary health systems.

Chan's Report challenges the idea that a mechanistic image of health care is adequate – one in which different disciplines live in different 'silos' and connect with each other in simple transactional ways. The image of a *living system* is also needed, where each component is a *cell* that has life of its own yet is also inter-dependent on other cells. The 'body' of primary health care needs dynamic interaction between different disciplines and organisations that results in mutual learning, trusted relationships and ongoing co-adaptation; and it all needs to come together at local, community level.

This book is about how to practically achieve this.

Are primary care and public health ready for comprehensive PHC?

Chan's 2008 WHO Report advocates 'reorganization of health services as primary care', and primary care should be the 'coordinator of a comprehensive response at all levels'. Doing this requires 'reforms that secure healthier communities, by integrating public health actions with primary care and by pursuing healthy public policies across sectors'.

The Report recognises that the best way to do this depends on the context. However, primary care in all contexts has recognisable strengths to work with:

* it provides a place to which people can bring a wide range of health problems
* it is a hub from which patients are guided through the health system
* it facilitates ongoing relationships between patients and clinicians, within which patients participate in decision-making about their health and health care; it builds bridges between personal health care and patients' families and communities
* it opens opportunities for disease prevention and health promotion as well as early detection of disease
* it requires teams of health professionals: physicians, nurse practitioners, and assistants with specific and sophisticated biomedical and social skills
* it requires adequate resources and investment, and can then provide much better value for money than its alternatives

To take a lead role in integrated health and care the primary-care team needs to become

a hub of coordination, effectively transforming the primary-care pyramid into a network, where the relations between the primary-care team and the other institutions and services are no longer based only on top-down hierarchy and bottom-up referral, but on cooperation and coordination.

(p. 55)

The need for community-based 'hubs of coordination' in health care is obvious. You would imagine that every country would develop them. However, Chan's Report gives only one example of a community hub of coordination working at scale – Cuba.

In the Cuban model, doctors work in multidisciplinary teams in comprehensive primary-care facilities. They are accountable for the health of a geographically defined population, provide both curative and preventive services, and work in close contact with their communities, social services, schools and other organisations (p. 65). Cuba is famous for its impressive health and literacy statistics, but it is also a small country (eleven million population) that has managed to insulate itself cleverly from forces that might damage its egalitarian vision. The Cuban model is desirable, but how to achieve it in other contexts needs some thought.

There are other, less established, examples of community-based hubs of coordination:

- Meads' 31-country study describes six ideal types of primary care organisation of which one, the 'community development agency', seems to be the kind of primary care hub of coordination envisioned by Chan. He writes 'Throughout such countries as Colombia, Bolivia, Peru, Brazil, Argentina and even parts of Canada (e.g. Quebec, Ontario), the community health centre or clinic is emerging as an engine driving forward participatory democracy' (p. 17) where participants maintain that 'health is a citizen, not a profession issue' (p. 100).

 Meads G. *Primary Care in the Twenty-First Century: an international perspective.* Abingdon: Radcliffe, 2006

Further analysis of Meads' work reveals that his six ideal types naturally cluster into three different kinds of community-based hubs of integration:

Model 1: Outreach franchise and polyclinic – integrating through medical practice
Model 2: Extended general practices and district health systems – integrating through multidisciplinary teams
Model 3: Managed care and community development agencies – integrating through networks, communities or systems

 Thomas, P., Meads, G., Moustafa, A., Nazareth, I. and Stange, K. Combined horizontal and vertical integration of care: a goal of practice-based commissioning. *Quality in Primary Care* 2008,16: 425–32

- *Community-oriented primary care* (COPC) includes community diagnosis, health surveillance and focused projects to improve the health of local communities. Kark gives case studies in urban Israel and rural South Africa.

 Kark, S.L. *The Practices of Community-Oriented Primary Health Care.* New York: Appleton-Century-Crofts, 1981

- Tudor Hart established a research and teaching general practice in Glyncorrwg, a South Wales village with a population of 5,000. Here he combined general practice and public health roles, using local data to identify health need and stimulate projects.

 Hart, J.T. *A New Kind of Doctor.* London: Merlin Press, 1988

- Liverpool, a UK city of half a million inhabitants, developed a *Healthy City 2000 Project* using the 'New Public Health' concept that emphasises community participation, health promotion and inter-sectoral collaboration. Alongside this, a strategic coalition developed general practice and broad-visioned primary care throughout the city.

Ashton, J. and Seymour, H. *The New Public Health*. Buckingham: Open University Press, 1988

Thomas P. Graver L. The Liverpool intervention to promote teamwork in general practice: an action research approach, Chapter 13 in P. Pearson and M. Spencer (eds) *Promoting teamwork in Primary Care: a research based approach*. London: Arnold, 1997, pp. 174–191

- In the UK there are signs of community-based coordinating hubs being developed at scale. In 2015 50 'Vanguard' sites were set up as a 'blueprint for the future of NHS and care services'. There are five kinds of these 'new care models':

1 Integrated primary and acute care systems (PACS) – joining up GP, hospital, community and mental health services
2 Multi-speciality community providers – moving specialist care out of hospitals into the community (MCP)
3 Enhancing health in care homes – offering older people better, joined-up health, care and rehabilitation services
4 Urgent and emergency care – new approaches to improve the coordination of services and reduce pressure on A&E departments
5 Acute care collaborations – linking hospitals together to improve their clinical and financial viability

New care models – supporting the design and implementation of new care models in the NHS. www.england.nhs.uk/ourwork/new-care-models/ (accessed 19 January 2017)

The potential of primary care to have a coordinated role for integrated care has long been recognised. Pioneering general practice after the inception of the UK National Health Service (NHS) led to the 1974 Leeuwenhorst European Study Group that created a consensus about the general practice/family medicine role that became accepted throughout Europe and is recognisable today. This states that general practice/ family medicine 'Makes efficient use of health care resources through co-ordinating care, working with other professionals in the primary care setting, and by managing the interface with other specialities, taking an advocacy role for the patient when needed', and 'Develops a person-centred approach, orientated to the individual, his/her family, and their community'.

Does comprehensive PHC conflict with professional training?

Everyone recognises the value of comprehensive primary health care. Its principles of person-centred, community-oriented care and coordinated health promotion are widely preached. One difficulty is that these terms can be interpreted in mechanistic, paternalistic and divisive ways, as well as vital, equal and inclusive ways. Another difficulty is the vital, equal and inclusive interpretation conflicts with basic pillars of professional training, including the nature of evidence, the meaning of health and even what it is to be an individual.

Historically, professionals and the public generally have been taught that positivist insights trump all other insights. This approach sees individual particles, like balls on a snooker table, so it is unable to illuminate complex or co-evolving situations. This leads to a static image of the world in which people are machines whose health will be improved by 'evidence-based' techniques. Complex human interactions are invisible to this way of seeing the world.

Modern understanding of paradigms of evaluation (Chapters 11 and 16) is much more holistic. It shows positivism to be merely one (very useful) way to illuminate phenomena; but others are equally valuable. A healthy person is a well-oiled machine and also a network of trusted relationships. The health of an individual has as much to do with the coherence of his or her life story as it does with objectively measured facts about their illnesses.

We must be realistic about how quickly this complex image of the world can be accepted. It replaces a sense of certainty in scientific knowledge with cycles of learning and change informed by scientific knowledge and other things. This kind of shift in thinking takes generations to achieve. We must go about this gently.

Medical and public health practitioners need to embrace a science of interactivity

Doctors do need a more sophisticated understanding of evidence and health and care. Chan's 2008 Report contains some disconcerting news that suggests that many doctors are not ready to take a meaningful role in developing healthy societies:

> Thus, person-centredness becomes the 'clinical method of participatory democracy', measurably improving the quality of care, the success of treatment and the quality of life of those benefiting from such care. In practice, clinicians rarely address their patients' concerns, beliefs and understanding of illness, and seldom share problem management options with them. They limit themselves to simple technical prescriptions, ignoring the complex human dimensions that are critical to the appropriateness and effectiveness of the care they provide.
>
> (p. 46)

Ouch!

We should not be surprised. Doctors are trained in the supremacy of positivist science and this leads to technical prescriptions. Not all doctors limit their work to this, nor all of the time, nor forever. And things are already changing. Even the term 'person-centred' is changing. If the new paradigm is an interactive one of multi-method inquiry, equality, participation and co-evolution, then the doctor–patient encounter is not strictly speaking 'patient-centred'. It is more Tuckett's notion of 'meetings between experts' – dialogue between patients and clinicians as equals helps them to make sense of sickness and health in the context of their life stories, and to negotiate actions to make those stories more coherent and more positive.

Tuckett, D. et al. *Meetings Between Experts: An Approach to Sharing Ideas in Medical.* Consultations Paperback. London: Routledge, 1985

GPs help patients to write positive, coherent life stories with a consulting style that Launer calls 'narrative-based primary care'. The clinician surfaces the array of issues that impact on the health and illness of patients and helps them to put them into better perspective. As Launer puts it, 'The job of a general practitioner is to help people to write better stories'.

 Launer, J. *Narrative-Based Primary Care: a practical guide.* Abingdon: Radcliffe Medical Press, 2002

Chan's call for 'reforms that secure healthier communities, by integrating public health actions with primary care and by pursuing healthy public policies across sectors' has implications for every aspect of society. It even informs what children learn at school and what modern-day citizens need to do to contribute to a healthy society. There is one urgent need – public health has to work with primary care. Primary care cannot take a population approach on its own.

In 2011 Hanlon et al. argued a need to reform public health practice to address issues of lifestyle and inequalities. This well-received paper described four previous 'waves' of public health practice. The authors argue a need for a fifth, with the following defining qualities:

1   Recognise that the public health community is dealing not with simple systems that can be predicted and controlled, but complex adaptive systems with multiple points of equilibrium that are unpredictably sensitive to small changes within the system.
2   Rebalance our mindset: from 'anti' (antibiotics, war on drugs, combating inequalities) to 'pro' (wellbeing, balance, integration), and from dominion and independence (through specialist knowledge and expertise) to greater interdependence and cooperation (the capacity to learn from and with others).
3   Rebalance our models: from a mechanistic understanding of the world and of ourselves as mechanics who diagnose and fix what is wrong with individual human bodies or communities, to organic metaphors where we understand ourselves as gardeners, enabling the growth of what nourishes human life and spirit, and supporting life's own capacity for healing and health creation.
4   Rebalance our orientation: integrate the objective (measurement of biological and social processes) with the subjective (lived experience, inner transformation) and inter-subjective (shared symbols, meanings, values, beliefs and aspirations).
5   Develop a future consciousness to inform the present, enabling innovation to feed the future rather than prop up the current unsustainable situation. Develop different forms of growth beyond the economic to promote high levels of human welfare.
6   Iterate and scale up through learning – a design process where we try things out, learn and share this learning. The major challenge of 'scaling up', which requires us to develop promising new approaches, should be taken as a

natural process of growth, driven by a desire to adapt and learn, rather than a mechanistic process that managers in large bureaucracies have responsibility for rolling out.

 Hanlon P., Carlisle, S., Hannah, M., Reilly, D. and Lyon, A. (2011) Making the case for a 'fifth wave' in public health. *Public Health*, 125(1): 30–6

In 2016 the UK Academy of Medical Sciences suggested a radical rethink of the public health role to address the 'complex array of interlinking factors that influence the health of the public'. The report suggests six key developments:

1 Rebalancing and enhancing the coordination of research
2 Harnessing new technologies and the digital revolution
3 Developing trans-disciplinary research capacity
4 Aligning perspectives and approaches
5 Working with all sectors of society
6 Engaging globally

The report recommends:

Better alignment between public health and clinical practice is needed if we are to retrieve the necessary shift to prevention. Our health and social care workforce must be equipped to understand the fundamental principles of 'health of the public' and the continuum of interventions from population to individual.

 Academy of Medical Sciences (AMS). Improving the health of the public by 2040: optimising the research environment for a healthier, fairer future. September 2016. https://acmedsci.ac.uk/snip/uploads/5807581429f81.pdf

The report did not explicitly mention primary care. Only the more generic 'clinical practice'. Perhaps this will come as they work out how to practically achieve 'better alignment'.

Community-oriented integrated care – the link, the glue, the cell

Since 1978 health-care integration in developed countries has focused particularly on care pathways for diseases. The value of broader integration for *health* has always been recognised, but never been realised at scale. Three reasons for this are:

1 *We lack a shared definition of health*. Diseases are things that we can focus on and treat. *Health* means living life forward, positively and optimistically. 'Dis-eases', as the name implies, may challenge health but their absence does not make someone healthy.
2 *We lack ways to evaluate complex things*. We use a laboratory approach, termed *positivism*. Shining positivism's light on complex situations reveals individual facts, but we need other lights to illuminate dynamic emergence. What we need is

fourth-generation evaluation, by which we combine positivism with *critical theory* and *constructivism.*
3   *We lack commitment to equal, positive relationships.* We fall into habits that stop us from seeing others as creative, loving beings. Instead we try to control them as objects. This stops us having playful adventures that build healthy communities. *Care plans* and *cycles of collaborative improvement* provide opportunities for shared 'adventures'.

These misunderstandings represent a deeper misunderstanding of how the past and the future relate to each other. More especially, we fail to see that simple certainty based on hindsight is no substitute for the complex co-adaptation needed to live life forwards. This complex co-adaption isn't simple at all. It means we have to weave together a range of insights and experiences to allow a coherent, collaborative future to emerge.

Unfortunately, too many of us believe that change happens as a simple consequence of knowledge or force. So we use 'carrots and sticks' to make people change. And we forget that people aren't donkeys. We tell, when we should listen. We force, when we should negotiate. We build new, when we should co-adapt. And we constantly forget *cognitive dissonance* – people will believe what they want to believe, not what is true.

So what should we do? Well, we can learn a few things from how jazz musicians improvise. Musicians listen to the beat and the melody, then offer new notes to enhance what others are playing. *They are responsive in the moment, playing to a shared beat, and co-creating a new tune.* This is how people develop a sense of 'we' from multiple 'I's. This is how trusted relationships form, how communities develop. It is how people learn and co-evolve.

This book proposes 'community-oriented integrated care' (COIC) as a way for primary care and public health to build community-based hubs of coordination for comprehensive PHC. COIC is the same things as community-oriented primary care (COPC) in that it brings together the functions of general practice and public health at local level to build communities for health. But it has three other features:

1   It focuses on geographic localities rather than individual practices – this allows different organisations to lead different kinds of health-promoting initiatives in synchrony.
2   It coordinates care pathways at locality (hub) level, making it easier to align various services that help people to live healthy lives out of hospitals.
3   It uses the *learning organisation* method of interlinked cycles of inter-organisational learning and change to help everyone to co-evolve.

The strengths of a community-based collaborating hub are revealed by three complementary images of connectivity:

1   A *link.* A link is a gateway to a care pathway. Each care pathway leads to different kinds of resource for different aspects of care and health promotion. Its strength is clarity – links can be monitored.
2   The *glue.* The glue is all the trusted relationships criss-crossing multiple boundaries and binding people together with a shared belief in 'public service ethos'. Its strength is resilience – if some ties break, others retain the overall shape.

3   A *cell*. A cell has a life of its own within the body of primary health care, and needs creative interaction with the rest of the body to remain alive. Its strength is innovation and adaptability – a cell can 'think for itself'.

These three images reflect Guba's three paradigms of inquiry (Chapter 16) and lead to different strategies for change:

1   A link, like post-positivism, sees direct connections and individual identities. Single particles and linear links makes change 'simple'. It's like balls hitting each other on a snooker table. This image expects change to happen directly from force.
2   The glue, like critical theory, sees hidden connections that tie people together. Multiple-way bonds makes change 'complicated'. It's like a machine. This image expects change to happen when everything moves at the same time.
3   A cell, like constructivism, sees co-adaptation and co-evolution. Co-evolution makes change 'complex'. It's like a living organism. This image expects change to happen when everything changes in response to changes in everything else.

All three of these images are needed to make COIC work.

How would you recognise COIC?

COIC includes *shared care* and *collaborative health promotion* at locality, community level. *Local* is important, because it's easier to see the range of factors that affect people's health when in their everyday, real-life situations. *Community* is important because it's easier to collaborate for a healthy society when people feel bound together with trusted relationships. If we step away from a local or community level, our focus narrows. For example in a hospital, the focus of attention is the reason for being there – usually treating a disease.

COIC does more than one thing at the same time. COIC makes it easier to treat diseases, through team-working between a huge numbers of community-based practitioners, and timely specialist input. Shared care, care plans, self-care and shared records all help to do this. Sometimes people with illnesses need to go to specialists, but specialist expertise can also be brought into local consultations through telephone, video and e-mail. This kind of team-working is sometimes called 'vertical integration'; its need is signalled in the 2016 NHS 'New Care Models' that integrate Primary and Acute Care Systems (PACS).

As well as treating diseases, COIC improves *health*. Being healthy means being able to build mutually supportive relationships that lead to healthy individuals, healthy families and healthy communities. This kind of team-working for a healthy society is sometimes called 'horizontal integration' and its need is signalled in the 2016 NHS 'new care models' of Multi-speciality Community Provider (MCP) that integrate care through locally based 'care hubs'.

COIC helps to integrate interventions that have nothing to do with general practice at all. Leadership teams from different organisations can lead cycles of collaborative improvement in the same local area. Over time, these cycles build teams, networks and communities for health and care within that area and gently challenge and embolden change in neighbouring areas – other 'cells' in the 'body' of primary health care.

A systems approach often develops naturally, as groups learn how to work well together – like putting dirty dishes on one side of the sink and clean on the other. But it usually happens in stuttering, unintegrated ways that do not sustain. The approach advocated here may do better by making clear the rationale and methods for long-term success.

Simple rules to achieve COIC

Simple rules remind individuals, organisations and networks how to integrate their work:

- Relate to the same geographic areas and seasons of activity.
- Participate in cycles of collaborative learning and coordinated change.
- See short-term goals as steps in longer-term journeys.
- Think of yourselves as being connected to others like organic cells in a body as well as mechanical links in a chain, united in a shared quest for whole society health.

Repeatedly doing these things produces a sense of belonging. A sense of community. It provides opportunities to have adventures with others that stimulate innovation, friendships and team-working. It models healthy behaviour – centred in the moment and alert to opportunities to do positive things; ready to trust, make leaps of faith and interact playfully with others; habitually listening to others and appreciating them. Mutuality, reciprocity, equality, generosity, appreciation – these are the values that these behaviours foster.

We must remember that the scale of change needed is enormous. COIC needs *everyone* to contribute to *connected communities* for health. All citizens should be *team players* who collaborate for health and care. So we must do what we can, patiently and persistently, in the company of others with a similar vision, until the time comes to hand over to others. Like gardeners, we need to consider ways to nurture every kind of flower. Like a relay team, none of us individually is solely responsible for success.

Incremental transformation into COIC

This book presents ways to achieve a collaborative culture in incremental and sustainable ways, using models that can be adapted to different contexts. You can practise the skills in small ways before you have to perform on a big stage. For example, *systems theory* allows you to envisage a system that has not yet been built; you can apply *organisational learning* in quiet safe places well before you develop a health community; you can practise *team-working* in everyday relationships long before you build *networks of high performing teams*.

Many people come across this kind of thinking too late. How can we expect citizens to trust emergent processes when compartmentalised, linear thinking is all that they have experienced? Trusted relationships lie at the heart of integration, but many people simply don't know how to build them – this book gives some pointers.

One last word from Margaret Chan's 2008 WHO Report:

> What eventually matters is the experience of patients accessing services. Trust will grow if they are welcomed and not turned away; remembered and not forgotten; seen by someone who knows them well; respected in terms of their privacy and dignity; responded to with appropriate care; informed about tests; and provided with drugs and not charged a fee at the point of service.
>
> (p. 108)

It is not just patients that need these things. We all need to be welcomed and remembered, respected and responded to with care. *And* we all need to welcome and remember, respect and care for others.

The book in brief

The book can be used as a manual – examples have considerable detail. It can be used as a textbook, providing both theory and models. But it is primarily a guide – every situation is different, so local reflection and piloting is needed before applying these ideas in yours.

There are five parts, each with four chapters. The first three discuss practical things that different leaders can do: policymakers (Part I), organisations such as general practices (Part II) and geographic localities (Part III). The last parts (IV and V) cover theory.

Part I: Policy to support integrated working

The image to support this part is *connected learning spaces*. In such places, people from different backgrounds can critique plans and review learning from pilot projects. Systems that enable learning between such spaces can create a learning system.

Chapter 1: Communities for health

Key message: To build communities for health, people need shared developmental spaces.

Chapter content: Localities of 30–70,000 population – *health networks* and *local health communities* – are a good 'village' size to build relationships within and between extended primary care teams that help everyone to integrate their ways of working.

Chapter 2: Shared care for long-term conditions

Key message: To develop trusted relationships within a local health community, people need valuable roles in integrated initiatives.

Chapter content: Most medical care for long-term conditions such as diabetes should happen in general practices (tier one). Tier two is a community-based clinic that supports tier one and aligns specialist teams to localities. Tier three is hospital care. Summaries of patient-held *care plans* are available to those who make ad hoc contributions.

Chapter 3: Seasons of learning and change

Key message: Spring, summer, autumn and winter help farmers to align ways of working. Four seasons of learning – *planning, coordinated actions, concrete experience and reflection* – help to align efforts for care, health promotion and quality improvement.

Chapter content: People from different parts of health care naturally do similar things between January and March, April and July, September and October, and November and December. These 'seasons' help to build a calendar of events for shared care, health promotion and participatory action research. Routinely gathered data help to evaluate the overall effect.

Chapter 4: Infrastructure of facilitation and communication

Key message: An infrastructure of facilitation and communication can support cycles of learning and change that integrate care and promote health.

Chapter content: *Applied research units* evaluate and maintain infrastructure to support annual cycles of inter-organisational reflection and collaborative improvement. They establish leadership teams, strategic partners, live manuals, stakeholder workshops, data gathering, publications and learning between case study sites.

Part II: Integrating care and promoting health from local organisations

The image to support this section is *interactive juggling*. Integrated care is too complex to directly control. There are too many things to do, and to know, to do it on your own. People need to meaningfully interact with others for their combined effort to be more than the sum of the parts. Networks of 'jugglers' can integrate activities across organisational boundaries. At the highest level jugglers do it 'blind' – they instinctively know where to throw things, and others know how to catch what they throw. It comes from years of practice and supportive infrastructure.

Chapter 5: Annual cycles of participatory action research

Key message: Annual cycles of collaborative inquiry and coordinated change support continuous quality improvements and integrated working. They can be led by locally based, semi-independent organisations such as general practices, pharmacies and schools.

Chapter content: Multidisciplinary leadership teams facilitate annual cycles of collaborative inquiry and coordinated change that align efforts for quality improvement inside and outside the organisation.

Chapter 6: Live manuals

Key message: When practitioners and managers from different parts of the system help to generate an information resource, the sense of ownership gained means that they are more likely to use the resource wisely.

Chapter content: A live manual is continually updated and practically used every day. It is where various leadership teams put the latest information, including educational updates and improvement projects, as well as explaining what different people need to do.

Chapter 7: How to see connections between parts and wholes

Key message: Leaders of community-oriented integrated care need images, theories and methods that help them to think clearly in complex situations.

Chapter content: The dynamic nature of community-oriented integrated care makes it difficult to know when to lead from the front and when from the back, when to take a principled stand and when to go with the flow, when to focus on detail and when to see bigger pictures. Images of complex creative activity help to find the right balance.

Chapter 8: How to run meetings that make sense of multiple perspectives

Key message: Community-oriented integrated care needs meetings at which people from different backgrounds learn from and with each other.

Chapter content: A good balance between shared stories and objective facts helps to make sense of different perspectives. This chapter describes techniques that help to do this in everyday meetings.

Part III: Integrating care and promoting health from geographic localities

The image to support this section is Case Studies of Local Health Communities. Case studies allow many different things to happen and the local story to be developed over time. Local health communities of about 50,000 population allow a sequence of research and improvement projects to take place. Routinely gathered quantitative data (e.g. hospital admissions and surveys) and qualitative data (e.g. patient stories) can build up rich pictures that help to witness the collective impact of multiple interventions on Wellbeing, Citizenship, Capacity and Economics. Learning between case studies helps to create good policy.

Chapter 9: Engaging people in cycles of inter-organisational learning and change

Key message: To develop a local community for health, multidisciplinary leadership teams in geographic areas need to engage large numbers of people in collaborative improvements.

Chapter content: Annual cycles of collaborative learning and coordinated action within geographic areas help *locality leadership teams* to engage a broad range of people in collaborative improvement projects that can incrementally build a local health community.

Chapter 10: Large group events help people to creatively interact

Key message: Stakeholder events help to build communities for health.

Chapter content: Established models of large group events engage large numbers of people of different backgrounds in collaborative learning and coordinated change.

Chapter 11: Structured inquiry – an important ingredient

Key message: Research, audits and service improvement projects influence local policy when they are embedded within annual cycles of locality improvement.

   Chapter content: Traditional approaches to research and development are inadequate for community-oriented integrated care. Fourth-generation evaluation, participatory action research and case studies are more appropriate because they can set inquiries within cycles of collaborative reflection and coordinated change.

Chapter 12: Maintain inner peace

Key message: To avoid losing sight of who you are within complex activity, leaders of community-oriented integrated care need strategies to maintain their inner peace.

   Chapter content: Create an island of sanity around yourself that allows you to see the woods and the trees in your own life, engage purposefully in whole system improvements and deal with grace with the misunderstandings of others.

Part IV: Understanding community-oriented integrated care

The image to support this section is a *human face*. The human face has features of both a machine and an organic, living system. *Machines* behave in predictable ways with clear links in a chain of actions. *Living organisms* co-create things through multiple-way interactions and learning from feedback loops. Both are needed.

Chapter 13: The story of community-oriented integrated care

Key message: Health-care systems throughout the world are moving towards community-oriented integrated care that emphasises team-working and local health communities.

   Chapter content: Community-oriented integrated care means that coordination of care and health improvements happens close to where people live. Care plans and local health communities help people to collaborate for shared care, self-care and healthy living.

Chapter 14: General practitioners are sense-makers

Key message: Community-oriented integrated care needs high-quality general practice.

   Chapter content: Primary care practitioners and managers see, more than others, different aspects of health and different contributions to care. They are well placed to orchestrate integrating activities. Patients have multiple problems and the most important often lurk below the surface. To address these, they think at several levels, repeatedly see people over time, bring hidden factors to the surface, and give patients things to think about and things to do. When issues arise that are beyond the knowledge of a practitioner, he or she finds the information through decision support mechanisms – within the consultation or before the next. This is how they cover the medical, surgical, social and mental health dictionaries.

Chapter 15: Health, identity and relationships

Key message: We need positive, holistic understandings of health, identity and relationships.

Chapter content: Health is being alive in the moment, able to reach out to and positively interact with others, forming networks of relationships that inform our identities. A healthy person rises above adversity to develop a coherent and positive life story – each person is the lead actor in the 'feature film' that is their life and co-actor in the 'films' of others. Health means that your life story is a story to be proud of. Refreshing relationships and having new adventures are needed to keep the story moving forwards and not become stuck in the past. Primary care practitioners help people to improve their stories in coherent and positive ways by helping them to use diseases as opportunities to improve resilience. They encourage people to seize opportunities of the moment to make good things happen.

Chapter 16: Three paradigms of inquiry illuminate evolving stories

Key message: Different approaches to inquiry reveal different things.

Chapter content: The success of laboratory (positivist) approaches to evaluation has marginalised approaches that reveal hidden connections and emerging phenomena. The result is a linear approach to change and a mechanistic approach to integration. It prioritises control over harmony, and fails to illuminate complex and evolving aspects of health. Guba has analysed three paradigms of inquiry that in combination can overcome this limitation. Together, *post-positivism*, *critical theory* and *constructivism* can see moving pictures. Through the lenses of post-positivism and critical theory you can see how individual part(icles) affect each other through simple and complicated interactions. Through the lens of constructivism you can see complex emerging phenomena and non-linear processes – an organic, living system.

Part V: Community-oriented integrated care – making it work

The image to support this section is *illuminating stories with complementary lenses*. On the left is the past. On the right is the future. Interactions in the present move a story on.

Chapter 17: Networks for complicated journeys

Key message: Community-oriented integrated care is a social movement *and* a machine

Chapter content: *Network theory* shows how to design a system that people can easily navigate and also have creative adventures within. An example is a railway network that shows how travellers can go to many different places and also align their travel plans with those of others. They need: a) nodes (stations and junctions) where different routes connect; b) timetables and maps; and c) trains that arrive on time. These are *mechanical aspects* of a network. They also need waiting rooms, restaurants and other places where passengers can interact with others, learn from them and review their travel plans. These are *living system* aspects. Integrated care needs both.

Chapter 18: Developing team players and systems thinkers

Key message: Everyone needs to be a team player and a systems thinker.

Chapter content: *Transactional analysis* shows how to interact creatively with others to develop trusted relationships. It highlights three 'ego states' – 'parent', 'adult' and 'child' – that we move between. When performing a functional task, like treating a disease, a one-dimension adult–adult or parent–child transaction is all that is needed. Human conversations that build trusted relationships require more sophisticated interactions. The person who initiates a conversation speaks from one ego state and signals the ego state he/she expects the other to respond with; that person responds accordingly and signals the ego state he/she expects in return, and so on. As long as each responds in the expected way, the interactions continue in what is called a 'game'. If someone responds in a different style, this 'crossed transaction' halts the conversation. A 'good game' concludes with a positive punch-line of 'I'm OK, you're OK' – conclusions have been negotiated; each demonstrates appreciation of the other; they have moved on their shared story. 'Bad games' diminish both/all players.

Chapter 19: Learning organisations build teams and communities

Key message: Organisations and systems as well as individuals need to continually learn and change.

Chapter content: *Organisational learning* theory shows how organisations as well as individuals can learn and change to transform whole systems. It shows how to develop learning communities. Learning organisations facilitate cycles of inter-organisational learning and change that include stakeholder events and collaborative improvement projects.

Chapter 20: Public health and primary care – an essential partnership

Key message: All citizens need to contribute to a healthy world.

Chapter content: This chapter describes how public health and general practice have important roles in reminding all citizens of their responsibilities to contribute to integrated care and health promotion, and align their work for health and care to the boundaries of local health communities. This includes families, schools, voluntary groups, universities, faith communities, local authorities, political parties and others. To engage in collaborative learning and coordinated change, citizens need a set of skills that should be learned and re-learned at all stages of life, especially at transformational moments.

Appendix

Skills to lead COIC are described under five learning aims:

1 Concepts for community-oriented integrated care (COIC)

    1.1 Trends in healthcare
    1.2 Three aspects of reality
    1.3 Creative interactions between different perspectives
    1.4 How organisations, networks and systems learn and change

2 Evaluating COIC

    2.1 Bring connections into view
    2.2 Assess team skills
    2.3 Research methods for transformational change
    2.4 Identify your own needs for personal transformation

3 Facilitating learning spaces

    3.1 Facilitate learning in groups
    3.2 Facilitate learning in a network
    3.3 Facilitate a large group event
    3.4 Bring dynamic interactions into view

4 Orchestrating whole system learning and change

    4.1 Lead system-transforming projects
    4.2 Build infrastructure that facilitates ongoing learning and change
    4.3 Manage coordinated sets of projects
    4.4 Feed-back useful data at appropriate times

5 Skills for personal balance

    5.1 Interact with others in ways that develop healthy stories
    5.2 Retain inner peace
    5.3 Maintain a network of personal and political support
    5.4 Maintain systems to manage information

Part I

Policy to support integrated working

In Part I:

Who might find Part I useful?

Image to support Part I: Connected learning spaces

Introduction to Part I: Community-oriented integrated care depends on trusted relationships

Box: Policy that supports community-oriented integrated care

Chapter 1: Communities for health. Localities of 30–70,000 population – *health networks* and *local health communities* – are a good 'village' size to build relationships between extended primary care teams that help everyone to integrate their ways of working.

Chapter 2: Shared care for long-term conditions. Most medical care for long-term conditions such as diabetes should happen in general practices (tier one). Tier two is a community-based clinic that supports tier one and aligns specialist teams to localities. Tier three is hospital care. Summaries of patient-held *care plans* are available to those who make ad hoc contributions.

Chapter 3: Seasons of learning and change. People from different parts of health care naturally do similar things between January and March, April and July, September and October, and November and December. These four 'seasons' help to build a calendar of events for shared care, health promotion and participatory action research. Routinely gathered data help to evaluate the overall effect.

Chapter 4: Infrastructure of facilitation and communication. *Applied research units* evaluate and maintain infrastructure to support annual cycles of inter-organisational reflection and collaborative improvement. They establish leadership teams, strategic partners, live manuals, stakeholder workshops, data gathering, publications and learning between case study sites.

Who might find Part I useful?

This part is primarily for policymakers, although others may also find it useful. It describes infrastructure to build and sustain local communities for health, and systems for shared care. These are needed to build *community-based coordinating hubs* that will help to realise the WHO concept of comprehensive primary health care – whole-society collaboration for whole population health. It also makes primary care more efficient.

This book advocates a participatory and systematic way to improve services that usually happens in more top-down and ad hoc ways. An annual calendar of events stimulates inter-organisational learning and change within and between *local health communities* – geographic areas of about 50,000 population. Clusters of general practices in these areas develop extended primary care teams and contribute to leadership of local initiatives in partnership with policymakers, public health, specialist services and many others.

Different local health communities pilot different things, led by local multidisciplinary *shared leadership teams*. An applied research unit supports them to lead the processes, evaluate outcomes and share learning. *Seasons* when everyone does similar things at the same time shape an annual calendar of linked events for *cycles of inter-organisational learning and change*. This fosters a development approach that is participatory and evolutionary. It enables local discussions that link local concerns with bigger pictures.

The approach considers people to be connected as though they are cells in the 'body' of health care, as well as components in a machine. If we want people from different parts of a system to integrate their efforts for care and health promotion we need more than mechanical linkage. Integration also requires us to build trusted relationships across disciplinary and organisational boundaries. 'Vertical' care pathways are not enough. We need 'horizontal' team-working between people of different insights too.

'Horizontal' team-working is needed for many purposes – patient care plans, co-design of services and health promotion campaigns, for example. Team-working is easier to achieve when people are aligned to the same geographic area – it is easier for everyone to get to know the others and align the plans of their organisations. In time, networks of relationships can become interwoven to create a sense of a local community – large numbers of people feel 'on the same side' ready to reinforce health messages, provide mutual support and collaborate for improvement projects. The best size of the area depends on the local situation. In UK cities, 50,000 is a good 'village' size – small enough to feel you belong and large enough to have political impact. But you have to consider your specific situation.

Geographic areas provide the opportunities for other organisations to lead initiatives in the same area that complement the effect of others; for example schools, faith groups, social services, voluntary groups. Merely acknowledging that they are contributing to a broader quest for whole-society health helps everyone to feel united. Each year different things happen depending on what different individuals and groups can manage.

Shared care, care plans and improvement projects emerge from this activity and provide opportunities for participants to develop their skills as team players. Shared leadership teams can improve their skills through learning sets and leadership courses. Networks of such teams can link with policy-making processes to make top-down and bottom-up initiatives enhance each other.

This part shows how to systematically develop and sustain infrastructure for integrated working at local level. Policy can chart a course to achieve this even in turbulent times. Keep your eyes focused on practical ways to apply the principles in your situation.

Image to support Part I: Connected learning spaces

This picture was drawn by Julian Burton (Delta7 Change Ltd – www.delta7.com) to portray the shared vision of a west London CCG.

Uncertainty is inevitable when improving health and integrating care, because everything is constantly changing in response to changes elsewhere. Unfortunately, uncertainty leads to anxiety in some people, causing them to disengage, obstruct or micro-control – behaviours that lead to poor outcomes.

Success comes from engaging with this complexity and acting at the right times to make progress that is, and feels, positive.

Trusting, learning spaces (the umbrellas) reduce anxiety by clarifying plans and sharing risk. They are more than places to coordinate activities. They include workshops where stakeholders critique plans and consider new developments. Facilitators help participants to learn from and with each other as they solve problems, share insights and generate improvement projects. The trust that is generated makes it possible to say things that might be considered 'undiscussable' – the 'elephants in the room'.

These workshops can be linked, so learning in one place can be considered in others. Events can be strategically linked to support *annual cycles of collaborative learning*

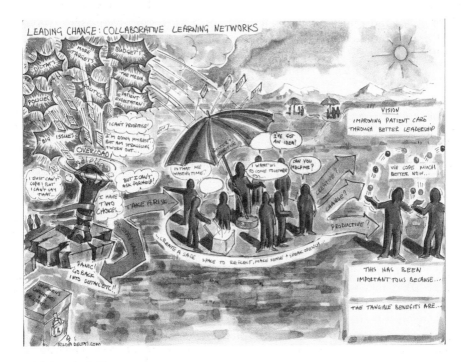

Figure 1 Connected learning spaces

and coordinated change that help local health communities to develop. Even more – different cycles of learning can link across much larger areas to enhance learning and influence, and create a culture of continual quality improvement. Scheduling workshops well in advance helps people to engage at appropriate times.

Introduction to Part I: community-oriented integrated care and health promotion depends on trusted relationships

Community-oriented integrated care (COIC) is shared care and collaborative health promotion at local, community level. At local level it is easier to see the large number of factors that affect someone's health. Further away, for example in hospital, conversations tend to focus on the reason for being there – usually an illness.

The secret ingredient of integrated care is a trusted relationship. You can get things done when the people you relate to (patients, professionals, neighbours, friends) react positively to you. Trust means that others will adapt their work to support yours, do the things they said they would, signpost resources you don't know about, give constructive criticism, and make honest assessments about whether they can add anything useful. Trusted relationships make people feel on the same side and more willing to join teams – work teams, leadership teams, strategy teams. In short, trusted relationships build teams that make things happen.

Trust develops when people work together to co-create good things. Annual cycles of inter-organisational reflection and coordinated action provide the opportunity to do this with large numbers of people. Multidisciplinary leadership teams facilitate these cycles and this encourages pilot projects and trusted relationships between their organisations. Ways to lead such cycles from single organisations like general practices or schools are described in Part II. Ways to lead them from geographic localities are described in Part III. Theories to guide success in any context are described in Parts IV and V.

To sustain COIC, relationships need to be repeatedly reinvigorated. Annual cycles of collaborative improvement within a geographic area help to do this. Localities of 30–70,000 population provide a good 'village' size for this. It is small enough to feel you belong, and large enough to have political effect. In health care, these localities are called 'health networks' when improving (medical) care pathways. They are called 'local health communities' when a broader alliance of community-based organisations collaborates for whole-population health. However, you need to assess your own situation – smaller and larger sizes may be more appropriate for you.

Success requires long-term vision and patience. An infrastructure of facilitation and communication is essential. Leaders need to understand the principles of organisational learning that bring change *more from helping people do things for themselves than from doing things to them*. It takes time to trust these processes, and even longer before they are used well. But when they become the normal way to operate, participants wonder how they ever did without them.

There are ways to speed up progress – faster cycles of change; adapting the model in response to learning of participants; using crises wisely; learning across case study sites. But progress might still feel slow, because it is organic – there has to be enough time for those who will have to live with the changes to feel that they 'own' them.

Your judgement matters here – go too fast and it will be slower overall; go too slow and people will get bored. Vary the speed as you get to know the territory.

Like a racing driver, accelerate–break–accelerate depending on the bends. It is easy to spin off the road at corners. And sometimes racing drivers need to go into the pits. Let it all settle. Give people time to think on their own. Give yourself a rest.

Policy that supports community-oriented integrated care

Policy throughout towns, cities and countries:

- Agree vision for inter-organisational collaboration for a healthy society, including public and private bodies, education, health, social and mental health care.
- Envision health as an aliveness of spirit that enables people to live life forwards with optimism, resilience and ecological awareness, as well as treating diseases.
- Form geographic localities of 30–70,000 population with the intention of developing integrated care and integrated health promotion within them.
- Provide incentives for localities to develop themselves as case studies of community-oriented integrated care, including health promotion as well as care for the sick.
- Support learning between case study sites, including connected workshops, shared projects, leadership courses and publications.
- Gather data to locality boundaries and evaluate effects on a) well-being, b) citizenship, c) capacity and d) economics.
- Provide training videos, manuals and courses to help people to become skilled at leading and evaluating annual cycles of inter-organisational improvement.
- Highlight the need at all stages of life for citizens to have adventures with those who are different from them, to learn from them and change as a consequence.

Policy within communities, networks and organisations:

- Maintain a database of organisations to collaborate in improvements, e.g. general practices, public health, community services, hospitals and intermediate care, local authorities, voluntary groups, businesses, schools, media, universities. Each should put forward three or more people of different disciplines as key contacts.
- Send a regular (e.g. monthly) interactive bulletin to key contacts in member organisations, inviting discussions about strategy and opportunities for collaboration.
- Facilitate a series of meetings, scheduled long in advance, for practitioners to interact creatively, e.g. for care plans, improvement projects and educational updating.

- Agree *seasons of care, seasons of health promotion* and *seasons of participatory action research* within annual cycles of inter-organisational learning and change, led by *shared leadership teams*.
- Develop multidisciplinary practice *leadership teams* within member organisations (e.g. general practices) to link their internal activities with external activities.
- Develop *system leadership teams* and *locality leadership teams* to coordinate cycles of improvement that stimulate integrated working.
- Provide courses for leadership teams, using principles of organisational learning that help participants to learn from and with each other.

Chapter 1

Communities for health

Key message: To build communities for health, people need shared developmental spaces.

In this chapter:

- Policymakers need to be fluent in the science of whole-system learning and change
- Geographic localities provide shared developmental spaces
- Cycles of learning and change can build communities
- Examples of community-building through cycles of learning and change:
  - Kark's Community-Oriented Primary Health Care
  - UK National Primary Care Facilitation Programme
  - Wales Teamcare Valleys
  - Health Education Authority team-building workshop programme
  - Liverpool local multidisciplinary facilitation teams
  - The King's Fund whole-system interventions
  - Southall Initiative for Integrated Care
  - West London Integrated Care Programme
  - New models of care and vanguard sites

- Infrastructure needs to support ongoing cycles of organisational learning and change
- Exercise: identify champions for change

Policymakers need to be fluent in the science of whole-system learning and change

In health care there are a vast numbers of things to do, and to know – more than any one discipline can know or do. To get everything done we need to maintain care pathways vertically and facilitate multidisciplinary team-working horizontally. We need to bring both together for shared care and collaborative health promotion. Shared developmental spaces that build communities for health are needed to do this.

Policymakers in health care mostly use the image of a *machine* to design integrated care, creating *hard systems* like care pathways that direct or control in 'linear' or 'vertical' ways. Part IV explains that the machine image is helpful for transactional tasks like treating an illness or referring into a care pathway, but does *not* help us with exploratory or complex things such as building relationships and leading a healthy life. For these, the machine image needs to be complemented by an organic *living system* image that brings into view the creative co-adaptations that happen when multiple factors interact in everyday life.

Living systems are dynamic in the organic way that a garden or seashore is dynamic. Many things happen at the same time, and everything adapts to the actions of others. They might be obeying the 'simple rule' (Chapter 16) of 'adapt or die'. The overall effect is like birds flocking – things move this way and that, then take off in unexpected directions (Chapter 16). When you are inside the 'flock', changing direction makes sense because you are caught up in the movement. This is how *cultural change* and *transformation* happen – everything changes seemingly as one through countless micro-adaptations.

Language and theories to describe this organic activity comes from many places, including *complexity theory, organisational learning* and *systems theories*. They all indicate that people should interact creatively across disciplinary and organisational boundaries. It has been called *boundary-spanning*. The overall effect of multiple boundary-crossing is what Stacey calls a *complex adaptive system* (Chapter 16) from which new things *emerge,* as though led by what Smith called an *invisible hand* (Chapter 16). Many find emergence and co-adaptation uncomfortable because they involve uncertainty and lead to unpredictable places. Many view them with suspicion because it conflicts with what they have been taught – linear, controlling models of change and laboratory understandings of research.

You are likely to encounter misunderstandings and self-doubt when applying these ideas because nothing is certain. To safeguard your own mental health you need to be fluent in theory, protected by a personal network of support and grounded in good practice.

Geographic localities provide shared developmental spaces

The power of teams to cause and sustain change has been known since the dawn of civilisation. Nevertheless, the idea that individuals should be the main agents of change and that change happens in direct, controlling ways has always been seductive – from ancient rulers and Machiavelli to modern-day individualism. In health care, the power of primary care teams to cause change is a twentieth-century awakening, as is explained in Chapter 18.

The strategic importance of networks and communities – *communities of practice* – is even newer. In 2004, Quebec set up 94 *local health networks* (LHNs) to improve service accessibility, continuity, integration and quality. Each LHN served a geographic area between 20,000 and 250,000 population. At the heart of each was a network of community health centres, long-term facilities for long-term conditions and (in 85 per cent) a hospital.

 Breton, M., Maillet, L., Haggerty, J. and Vedel, I. (2014) Mandated Local Health Networks across the province of Québec: a better collaboration with primary care working in the communities? *London Journal of Primary Care,* 6: 4, 71–78, DOI: 10.1080/17571472.2014.11493420

In 2005 Staffordshire (UK) developed a local health community in which four primary care trusts worked in partnership with hospital, community, social and ambulance services.

 North Staffordshire Local Health Community Integrated Service Improvement Plan 2005/06 to 2007/08. http://webarchive.nationalarchives.gov.uk/20091107211958/ http://www.combined.nhs.uk/nsPortal/cmsitem?documentPath=NSLib/ISIP%20 (2005-06%20to%202007-08)&version=1.

In 2009 the NHS Integrated Service Improvement Programme (ISIP) described *local health communities* as a key long-term strategy:

> The NHS Integrated Service Improvement Programme (ISIP) is working with Strategic Health Authorities to underpin the change agenda by supporting local health communities (LHCs) with delivery of service transformation . . . These are not pilots, the expectation is that they will have transformed delivery of care, at pace, and will be operating new models of both commissioning and provision.

 ISIP Local Health Community demonstrator sites. http://webarchive.national archives.gov.uk/20090218170434/http://www.networks.nhs.uk/networks. php?pid=634

In 2014, general practices in UK cities started to cluster into geographic areas of about 30–70,000 population. Each was thought of as a 'village' within larger towns and cities to provide a *shared developmental space* for people to learn from and with each other, pilot innovation and align their efforts for integrated care and health promotion. We can think of them as 'cells' within the 'body' of health care.

Some GPs used these 'cells' to share services, for example out-of-hours cover, calling them *health networks* to indicate collaboration between health-care professionals. Others used them to engage local authorities and communities in strategic developments, and called them *local health communities* to indicate broader collaboration for whole-population health.

Larger groupings of general practices ('GP Federations') formed at the same time to oversee development as service *providers*. Many shared the same geographic boundaries as clinical commissioning groups that *buy* services, and also with local authority boroughs that provide *social care*. They are meant to provide the architecture to support whole-system integration.

The intention for local health communities to be a long-term investment was signalled in 2015 when fifty *vanguard sites* were chosen throughout the UK to 'join up GP, hospital, community and mental health services'.

 https://www.england.nhs.uk/ourwork/futurenhs/new-care-models/

Cycles of learning and change can build communities

Local health communities challenge the ideas that only individuals lead change, and that change happens in straight lines. They remind us that trust is more co-created than forced, and that it emerges from healthy human interaction. How to facilitate this is a contested question – and the central theme of this book. 'The body of knowledge on networks is still emerging', according to a 2013 review of networks in health care.

The Health Foundation. *Leading Networks in Healthcare: learning about what works – the theory and the practice.* www.health.org.uk/publication/leading-networks-healthcare

A geographic locality is only one way to develop a community for health. Health care is only one institution to lead health improvements. Schools, faith groups and clubs of all kinds have networks of members who can be mobilised to work for the health of society, as well as the particular interest that defines that group. They too can use images of machines and living system in combination. They too can apply principles of organisational learning.

Building trusted relationships within a community or network is not straight forward. Trusted relationships are slow to build and can be easily destroyed by thoughtless actions. Mechanisms to develop and refresh relationships are always needed. Calling a locality a *local health community* is a start. It raises expectations that the group will operate in a way that makes its effect more than the sum of its parts. But interventions, leadership and practical support are needed for this potential to be realised.

The approach advocated here is *annual cycles of inter-organisational improvement* within and between localities. The cycles are led by multidisciplinary leadership teams – *practice leadership teams* within general practices, *locality leadership teams* within local health communities and *system leadership teams* that extend to all parts of a system.

Theories to help understand the approach are covered in Parts IV and V:

- Community-oriented integrated care is important and feasible (Chapter 13)
- Generalist and specialist practitioners have complementary roles (Chapter 14)
- People grow together through shared adventures (Chapter 15)
- Different paradigms of knowledge are needed to reveal co-creativity (Chapter 16)
- Systems have both mechanical and organic features (Chapter 17)
- Trusted relationships come from playing 'good games' (Chapter 18)
- Learning organisations help both groups and individuals to learn (Chapter 19)
- Everyone in society needs to contribute (Chapter 20)

PAUSE: How do you develop the communities to which you belong?

Examples of community-building through cycles of learning and change

The need to develop communities for integrated care and integrated health promotion finds its roots in the 1978 World Health Organization international agreement (Chapter 13) that all citizens need to contribute to healthy communities. Strategy to achieve this in the NHS has changed since 1978 from controlling 'top-down' targets towards cycles of learning and co-design for integrated working. This shift is illustrated by the changing language in the following examples.

Kark's Community-Oriented Primary Health Care

Kark's 1981 analysis of *community-oriented primary health care* illustrates how strategy of the time was structural – health centres provided services and treated 'clinical syndromes':

The move towards a union of the previous separate preventative and curative services (hospital services, public health practice and primary health care) was reflected in various proposals after World War 1 . . . among the cornerstones of these proposals was the comprehensive health center [p. 9] . . . Primary care includes curative and preventive personal services . . . extending to include mental health services, preventive cardiology, and health care for the aged and disabled [p. 15] . . . [Including] participation of individual patients in decision making . . . Perhaps the most important prerequisite for satisfactory functioning of a community in its own health care is a relationship of basic trust between the community and the health team [p. 19]. Diagnosis of the state of health of a community is important [p. 25] . . . regarding health as a state of wellbeing and not merely the absence of disease is essential [p. 26] . . . the concept of wellbeing, or healthiness, including the subjective feeling of wellbeing, soundness of body and mind, and social functioning consistent with expected roles in society [p. 28] . . . the concept of a *clinical syndrome* is essential to clinical diagnosis [and also to] community diagnosis [that] involves finding an association between various states of health in a community [p. 31].

 Kark, S.L. *Community-Oriented Primary Health Care*. London: Appleton-Century-Crofts, 1981

UK National Primary Care Facilitation Programme

The primary care facilitator was developed in 1982 to help general practices develop Kark's vision. By 1994 there were 304 in the UK. They helped practices to develop well-man clinics that screened for risk factors for heart disease. The National Primary Care Facilitation Programme oversaw the network of facilitators. A national steering group considered feedback from all parts of the UK. This led many to sense the need for more dynamic initiatives that helped people to help themselves. They used the language of *learning* – 'adult learning', 'work-based learning', 'action learning', 'organisational learning'. For example, in Sheffield an initiative called Towards Coordinated Practice caused city-wide change by helping general practices to reflect on comparative data and plan their own developments.

 Wilson, A. *Changing Practices in Primary Care: a facilitator's handbook*. London: Health Education Authority, 1994

Welsh Teamcare Valleys

The idea that cycles of learning and change would cause sustainable change was illustrated by Teamcare Valleys. Between 1990 and 1993, 36 fellows were appointed by the University of Wales. They worked in multidisciplinary teams to support general practices in deprived areas of South Wales to improve services. Through audits, improvement projects, training and discussions, they stimulated a 'hive of argument, discussion and planning' (p. xviii).

 Bryar, R. Teamcare Valleys: a multifaceted approach. Chapter 5 in P. Pearson and M. Spencer (eds), *Promoting Teamwork in Primary Care: a research based approach*. London: Arnold, 1997

Health Education Authority team-building workshop programme

This programme flowed naturally from the growing awareness that *team-learning* stimulates team-working and integrated working. 1989 saw the launch of the Health Education Authority *Primary Health Care Team Workshop Strategy for Disease Prevention and Health Promotion*. At each two-day residential workshop, five multidisciplinary practice teams devised plans for health promotion for their practices. Pre- and post-workshop meetings helped the practice teams to translate their plans into action. An inter-organisational 'Local Organising Team' planned and led the workshops. Evaluation showed this approach to be 'a very effective mechanism for the enhancement of prevention and health promotion in general practice' (p. 52). This initiative highlighted the need for networks of leadership teams that span organisations to facilitate change, and not merely projects.

  Spratley, J. *Joint Planning for the Development and Management of Disease Prevention and Health Promotion Strategies in Primary Care*. London: Health Education Authority, 1991

Liverpool local multidisciplinary facilitation teams

Different cities in the UK adapted the Health Education Authority team-building workshops to support locally designed initiatives. In 1992 in Liverpool, the workshops were used to develop *local multidisciplinary facilitation teams* that facilitated general practice development in geographic areas of 70,000 population. This initiative concluded that evaluation of complex interventions in primary care (such as theirs) required (p. 187):

- A participatory action research approach
- Participation of diverse stakeholders
- A multidimensional evaluation framework

This project illustrated a growing awareness of the need to stimulate cycles of learning and change in all organisations and throughout whole systems, year on year.

  Thomas, P. and Graver, L. The Liverpool intervention to promote teamwork in general practice: an action research approach. Chapter 13 in P. Pearson and M. Spencer (eds), *Promoting Teamwork in Primary Care: a research based approach*. London: Arnold, 1997, pp. 174–191

The King's Fund whole-system interventions

These interventions facilitated learning and integration throughout whole systems by creating partnerships for health in UK cities. They enabled people from many different sectors to co-design integrated systems of care, using methodologies of Future Search, Open Space and Real Time Strategic Change (described in Chapter 16).

  Pratt, J., Gordon P. and Plamping, D. *Working Whole Systems: putting theory into practice in organisations*. London; King's Fund, 1999

Southall Initiative for Integrated Care

City-wide initiatives can lose contact with grassroots practice. So between 2009 and 2012 the Southall Initiative for Integrated Care explored ways to combine locally based communities for health with whole-system learning and change. Twenty-three general practices took part, clustered into four localities each of about 15–20,000 population.

 Evans, L., Green, S., Sharma, Kiran, Marinho, F. and Thomas, P. (2014) Improving access to primary mental health services: are link workers the answer? *Journal of Primary Care*, 6: 2, 23–28, DOI: 10.1080/17571472.2014.11493409

This initiative used five mechanisms:

- **An annual cycle of collective reflection and coordinated action:** A sequence of events was scheduled long in advance. They allowed stakeholders from different organisations to a) agree shared vision and priorities for improvement, b) devise and lead coordinated improvement projects and c) consider learning from the projects.
- **Inter-organisational shared leadership teams:** The leadership teams engaged people from their own organisations and disciplines in improvement projects that emerged from the annual cycle of activity.
- **An overt expectation that membership of shared leadership teams would change each year:** Organisations concerned with mental health, acute care, social care and community care contributed to annual cycles of collective reflection and coordinated action. Each year they allocated different people to the multidisciplinary project leadership teams.
- **Clustering of general practices into geographical areas:** Leadership teams in each area led developments on behalf of larger areas.
- **Routinely gathered data about cost and quality of care within the GP clusters:** The data helped to monitor the impact of the collaborative activity.

West London Integrated Care Programme

In 2012 the West London Integrated Care Pilot (ICP) began in the eight local authority boroughs of west London. The ICP revolved around monthly case conferences within fifty geographic areas of approximately 50,000 population. They were called 'health networks' and they hosted multidisciplinary group meetings (MDGs).

Ealing highlighted five mechanisms in its version of the ICP:

1 Staff employed by community services and the local authority were attached to the boundaries of Ealing's seven health networks, creating extended primary care teams; two co-chairs in each area (14 in total) led collaborative improvements that included these attached staff
2 Practitioners from different disciplines and organisations were paid to attend the MDGs to discuss the care of patients who needed multiple agency input (especially those with diabetes or who are elderly)
3 Participants at the meetings also devised innovations to improve whole systems of care (there was an Innovation Fund to apply for funds)

4   Care plans were developed for patients at risk of hospital admission.
5   Practices were paid to develop care plan for elders and people with diabetes.

 Unadkat, N., Evans, L., Nasir, L., Thomas, P. and Chandok, R. (2013) Taking diabetes services out of hospital into the community, *London Journal of Primary Care*, 5: 2, 87–91. DOI:10.1080/17571472.2013.11493386

New models of care and vanguard sites

In the UK, the 2015 vanguard sites for the *new care models* programme showed a shift of strategy for health-care planning towards cycles of learning and co-design for integrated working. It is 'one of the first steps towards delivering the Five Year Forward View', intended to 'develop a blueprint for the future of the NHS and care services'. By 2016, 50 vanguard sites were set up with values of *clinical engagement, patient involvement, local ownership* and *national support*. They were expected to co-design integrated working in five areas:

- Integrated primary and acute care systems – joining up GP, hospital, community and mental health services
- Multi-speciality community providers – moving specialist care out of hospitals into the community
- Enhanced health in care homes – offering older people better, joined-up health, care and rehabilitation services
- Urgent and emergency care – new approaches to improve the coordination of services and reduce pressure on A&E departments
- Acute care collaboration vanguard sites

 NHS England. New care models: vanguards – developing a blueprint for the future of NHS and care services. September 2016. https://www.england.nhs.uk/ourwork/futurenhs/new-care-models/

Infrastructure needs to support ongoing cycles of organisational learning and change

Within 30 years, strategy for integrated care and health promotion has shifted from outreach from health centres to treat diseases, towards co-design of environments for shared care and health promotion, using cycles of learning and change to build local health communities.

The policy 'shift' is more a changed balance:

- Treating diseases still matters, but policymakers also recognise the value of building system-wide integration, and helping people to help themselves.
- Top-down targets, models from other places and bottom-up pilot projects still have their place, but policymakers also recognise the value of networks of leadership teams to stimulate discussions about locally relevant strategy for health and care.
- Individual treatments still matter, but policymakers also recognise the value of shared care and the complementary strengths of specialists and generalists.

Strategy to move this agenda forwards appeals to a science of whole-system learning and change (Parts IV and V). This means broadening our understanding of learning to see learning as more than an individual pursuit. *Organisations, networks* and *systems* can also learn; like individuals they need cycles of reflection and action (Chapter 19).

Success requires applying principles of *organisational learning* throughout whole systems. How to do this is unfamiliar to many – understandably since this is not taught at school or medical school. To make understandable complex processes of whole-community learning and change it helps to describe *packages* of activity that can be linked to stimulate continuous quality improvements throughout the system.

Here are some 'packages' that help whole-system learning and change:

1   **Shared developmental spaces:** geographic areas where people can incrementally build local communities for health
2   **Annual cycles of inter-organisational learning and change:** linked events, scheduled long in advance, that engage people in collaborative projects
3   **Projects:** with valuable short-term outcomes that contribute to longer-term aims
4   **Networks of leadership teams:** supported by leadership courses to develop their abilities to act in synchrony and continually improve
5   **Data:** routinely gathered, to evaluate the combined effect of coordinated actions within geographic areas on a range of outcomes including well-being, citizenship and capacity, as well as economic

Exercise: identify champions for change

Identify individuals, groups and networks in your case study that are ready to take a fuller role in developing community-oriented integrated care. Consider ways to connect their activities with those of others in your case study. What projects might they lead?

Chapter 2

Shared care for long-term conditions

Key message: To develop trusted relationships within a *local health community*, people need valuable roles in integrated initiatives.

In this chapter:

- Three-tier model of shared care for long-term conditions
- Shared records
- Care plans

    o   What is a care plan?
    o   What should a care plan include?
    o   Who might benefit from a care plan?

- Packages of care
- Exercise: create a care plan

Three-tier model of shared care for long-term conditions

Community-oriented integrated care challenges the common expectation that long-term conditions should be treated in hospitals by specialists. Instead they should be treated in primary care clinics as far as possible, with timely specialist input. A good example is the three-tier model of care for diabetes piloted in west London.

 Unadkat, N., Evans, L. Nasir, L. Thomas, P. and Chandok, R. (2013) Taking diabetes services out of hospital into the community, *London Journal of Primary Care*, 5: 2, 87–91, DOI:10.1080/17571472.2013.11493386

Each general practice develops its own (tier one) nurse-led diabetes clinic. General practices cluster into geographic localities of 30–70,000 population – termed *health networks* (for medical care) and *local health communities* (when collaborating for community-based health promotion). All practices in these localities use the same (tier two) diabetes clinic based in a community clinic and run by a team of diabetes specialist nurses and consultants. The tier-two team sees patients from that health network (when needed), and also provides support to primary care clinicians. This support includes telephone and email advice and educational updating. Hospital care (tier three) is reserved for patients who need multiple consultant input, have brittle diabetes and children.

Data about diabetes control and use of health care are routinely gathered by practices and health networks. Each year a cycle of learning and service improvement includes three or four stakeholder events at which practitioners and managers from different health networks compare data and co-design service improvements.

Lessons from one system of care (e.g. diabetes) are used to design others (e.g. mental illness or respiratory diseases).

This chapter describes how the three-tier model, coupled with shared records, care plans and packages of care, can build teams throughout care pathways.

PAUSE: Think of a system of care for a long-term condition that you know (for example diabetes). In what ways does it stimulate shared care?

Shared records

Practitioners in the three-tier model of care for long-term conditions need shared records. Patients, specialist and generalist practitioners all need to be able to update them.

Shared records have long been used for pregnant women and people with diabetes. The patient has a hand-held record that they take to different practitioners. Modern computer systems make it possible for members of a shared care team to see records electronically.

Electronic records also allow ad hoc contributions to care plans, for example by out-of-hours practitioners. This service originated to manage overnight emergencies, but has gradually taken on other responsibilities, including 111 telephone advice, unscheduled care ('walk-in') centres, night nurses and general practices attached to A&E departments. Increasingly this service attracts 'portfolio' GPs who have roles in different parts of the system and are skilled at switching between consulting styles appropriate for planned and emergency care.

Out-of-hours services could develop in partnership with health networks and local health communities. The aim would be to continue into the night and weekends the care planning and health promotion activities started during the day. The practitioners involved would become temporary members of extended primary care teams.

For example, the notes of patients with care plans could be flagged to enable the out-of-hours GPs to see what needs to be done beyond the complaint of that moment. This might mean encouraging a patient to continue their plan for the year, or record their blood pressure, or be faithful to their advance directives (e.g. whether or not to resuscitate or transfer to hospital). The out-of-hours GPs could send information to daytime GPs that might be useful (e.g. information about an impromptu family conference that took place at a weekend). Similarly, daytime services could provide out-of-hours services with a database of local health promotion services, and encourage patients to use them.

Out-of-ours services could develop portfolio doctors as 'system walkers' who understand the constraints and potentials of different kinds of primary care practice. They could develop strategic partners for education and research that enable clinicians and managers to lead system-wide evaluated improvements. They could gather data about patient contacts to inform commissioning decisions. All of these steps are helped by shared records.

Care plans

What is a care plan?

A care plan summarises a patient's illnesses and plans for the year. For example, someone with diabetes could have a plan for exercise, home monitoring, annual blood tests and eye checks. As well as providing useful overview, the care plan provides an agenda for action that is shared between patients, their families, and health and social care practitioners in the shared care team. Patients hold their own care plans and they can be made available electronically to others who contribute to their care, subject to confidentiality safeguards.

Between 2012 and 2014, in west London, primary care practitioners in health networks (geographic areas of about 50,000) met regularly to co-create care plans for patients with complex needs (e.g. frail or elderly). Consultant physicians, mental health specialists, social workers and district nurses also attended these meetings and contributed to the care plans. Over time, mutual learning and shared projects resulted in trusted relationships between participants, and this became transmitted to their various disciplines, improving relationships beyond the people in the room. Care plans became 'grit in the oyster' – they provided a focus for practitioners from different organisations to get to know each other.

What should a care plan include?

Include in a care plan:

- A brief description of their life story, including their medical conditions, goals for well-being, ongoing care and advance directives.
- Medications (name, frequency, dose).
- Negotiated action points for that year (e.g. exercise, self-monitoring, self-help, relationship building, new interests).
- List of key contacts, especially the shared care team including carers (e.g. the neighbour who has a back-door key), next of kin and other significant people.

Care plans are meant to help others to quickly see a brief summary of everything, so they can contribute useful things in a timely way. They are not meant to say everything, so:

- Keep care plans brief.
- Agree where they will be found in the notes and always put them in this place.
- Write care plans in simple English.
- Keep large amounts of data away from care plans (you can point to where they are).
- List dates of significant events (e.g. medication review).

A simple care plan

Story: Mr Smith is a 69-year-old retired school teacher (born 19XX) who has had non-insulin dependent diabetes since 2010 and hypertension since 2014. Both are well controlled and require only annual review at the practice (July).

He lives with his wife in their family home. Two of their four children live nearby and one or other visits most weeks. He is a keen gardener. He has no advance directives.

Medications: XXX

Action Plan: He aims to go for a walk to the park each day, go dancing once a week, maintain his garden and help at a local charity shop. He will monitor his blood pressure at home once a month.

Key Contacts: XXX

PAUSE: What do you think a care plan should include, and why?

Who might benefit from a care plan?

People who have a long-term condition of any kind (e.g. diabetes, asthma, cancer) benefit from a care plan that reminds everyone what needs to be done and when. Care plans are especially important for those who are at high risk of admission to hospital.

Risk stratification tools help to decide who is at risk of admission to hospital. They analyse patients by age, medical conditions and previous use of the health services to score their likelihood of hospital admission.

Risk stratification tools are limited. They do not take account of local insights into reasons for a patient to seek hospital care. They also do not take account of patients who would benefit from a care plan yet are not at high risk of admission to hospital. If a practitioner is paid for care plans, they should negotiate the ground rules for the use of their local knowledge for such patient (e.g. writing in the patient's notes the perceived need for a care plan).

As well as reminding about routine monitoring, care plans provide opportunities for thoughtful discussions between practitioners and patients. Consider the following scenarios, each of which deals with a specific problem, and at the same time opens out a conversation about health improvements:

- At annual update of a care plan the clinician might say: 'Here is the summary of your medical problems and home circumstances. Now let's talk about what you would like to do in the coming year to improve your overall health. From what you have said you are happy to continue doing home monitoring for your diabetes and blood pressure, and also the lifestyle routine you worked out last year. What else would you like to do to improve your overall health – for example, new interests, advance directives . . .?'

- At a meeting of the extended primary care team to review care plans, a team member might say: 'We have reviewed the care plans, identified new people to join the case management register and heard about some new services that may help our frail elderly. What else is emerging that may improve the overall health of our community – new illnesses, local concerns, festivals . . .?'
- In an out-of-hours consultation, as well as dealing with the immediate concern, the clinician might say: 'I see in your care plan that you monitor your blood pressure? May I see the readings? Do you want me to tell your daytime GP that you are getting side-effects from these tablets and enjoying your dance classes . . .?'

Packages of care

From time to time there will be a need for particular interventions. Locally agreed formats will be available:

- *Family conferences* – to develop a whole family plan for care
- *Advanced directives* – to agree whether to resuscitate and preferred place to die
- *Mental capacity* – to decide whether a patient is fit to make decisions
- *Power of attorney* – to permit another person to make decisions for a patient
- *Regular review* – care plan update and long-term condition clinics

Exercise: create a care plan

Sit down with someone (e.g. a patient or friend) and create a care plan for them. In what ways was this valuable?

Chapter 3

Seasons of learning and change

Key message: Spring, summer, autumn and winter help farmers to align ways of working. Four seasons of learning – *planning, coordinated actions, concrete experience* and *reflection* – help to align efforts for care, health promotion and quality improvement.

In this chapter:

- Cycles of learning and change can harmonise top-down and bottom-up plans
- Seasons of care and health promotion can align the plans of different organisations
- Seasons of participatory action research can support learning and change
- What happens in each season?
- Routinely gathered data can evaluate case studies of integrated care
- Real-time strategic change
- Exercise: identify relationship-building activities

Cycles of learning and change can harmonise top-down and bottom-up plans

Top-down control can force people to align their activities, but in doing this it often stifles bottom-up creativity. Bottom-up community development can facilitate local team-working and innovation, but in doing this it can inhibit learning from other places. Both top-down and bottom-up approaches are needed for whole-system harmony.

This presents the strategic question: 'What strategy can achieve top-down control, bottom-up innovation, and whole system harmony at the same time?'

The answer presented in this book is: 'Seasons of care that frame annual cycles of collaborative learning and coordinated change.'

Practitioners and managers from different parts of the system attend events that allow them to listen to others, negotiate the best ways forward and adapt their ways of working to fit well together. Participants often come to see that top-down policy and bottom-up innovation can complement each other with a bit of lateral thinking and a collaborative spirit.

A natural annual timetable affects most health-care organisations. People like to go on the big annual holidays (August and December) with work completed and a plan ready for when they come back (September and January). Most organisations provide an end-of-year report in April, making the January to March period a period of data gathering and planning for the coming year. Most organisations know their annual budgets in April, making this a good time to finalise plans. The Quality Outcomes Framework (QOF) requires care plan updates from April each year making this a good to time to do the bulk of care plan updates.

These dates shape four natural 'seasons' when people naturally do similar things:

January–March: Season of planning – gather data for annual reports and future plans
April–July: Season of coordinated actions – start the annual cycle of activity
August–October: Season of concrete experience – focus on getting the work done
November–December: Season of reflection – 'unfreeze': stand back to review learning

An annual calendar of collaborative learning and coordinated change events can be set onto these seasons that engages stakeholders from many different disciplines and organisations.

PAUSE: How do you align the activities of various organisations in your case study?

Seasons of care and health promotion can align the plans of different organisations

Care is important. It means reaching out to help someone who has a need. Sometimes care is reactive – when someone becomes ill you care for them. Sometimes it can be planned, for example seasonal illnesses like influenza in the cold months and hay fever in the warm.

Health promotion is different from care. It means building environments and providing activities that help people to help themselves to live healthy, meaningful lives.

Care plans for people with long-term conditions like diabetes, dementia and mental illness are commonly updated on people's birthdays. This has the advantage of spreading activity throughout the year. However it makes it difficult to align activities for care and health provided by different organisations.

Bunching care-plan updates into times of year has the advantage of aligning the activities of different organisations for both care and health promotion. For example, health promotion courses to understand diabetes self-care can happen at the same time as media campaigns to understand diabetes and with diabetes care plan updates.

Seasons of participatory action research can support learning and change

Combined caring and health promotion is still not enough. It is also important to know what models are most likely to be effective. This is not always obvious. Some practitioners will tell you that at times the most caring thing to do is not to care! Generating this kind of knowledge and acting on it is the role of *research and development* (R&D).

The term R&D is often interpreted to mean laboratory research, where knowledge is generated in one place and then simply 'rolled out' elsewhere. This approach is called the paradigm of *positivism*. Chapter 16 explains why this is *not* helpful to evaluate complex and dynamic things. Instead a combination of paradigms – positivism, critical theory and constructivism – helps to see different aspects of the whole.

Chapter 11 describes fourth-generation evaluation that can bring together different paradigms of inquiry, and *participatory action research* (PAR) as a way to achieve it. PAR combines inquiries with a sequence of opportunities for local people to reflect on data in the light of their experiences, and pilot improvements. The breadth of insight, sense of ownership and pilot testing helps to find the best next steps.

PAR is one of a family of approaches to R&D that combines evidence with local discussion and coordinated action for change. Other approaches include *real-time strategic change*, *action science*, *case studies*, *collaborative inquiry*, *appreciative inquiry* and *experience-based co-design*. These approaches all recognise that the certainty of the past is different from the uncertainty of living life forwards – so you have to look at things from different perspectives and test ways to get the best fit with the local context. They recognise that:

- Evidence generated in one context is not necessarily relevant to another because local factors are different.
- Sudden interventions can disrupt local balance and actually worsen things.
- The more a situation is complex, the greater is the need for a PAR-type approach that nests knowledge generation within processes of local learning and change.

Seasons of care, seasons of health promotion and seasons of participatory action research can be integrated through an annual cycle of activity.

What happens in each season?

Seasons of care, health promotion and participatory action research can frame annual cycles of collaborative learning and coordinated change within which participants enhance each other's contributions. Of course, reactive work happens all the time – managing new problems and updating plans are not purely seasonal.

January–March: season of planning

For care: This is the time of year when everyone tidies up one year and prepares for the next in time for the end of year report. They gather data and provide training arising from the past year's development. This is a good time to plan the detail of strategy for the year.

    For health promotion: This is a good time to plan health-promotion campaigns for the year.

    For PAR: This is a good time for practices, supported by external agencies, to conduct rapid appraisals to plan the coming year's improvement project(s).

April–July: season of coordinated actions

For care: This is a good time to do the bulk of annual care-plan updates. Patients and partner agencies (e.g. out-of-hours services) can hold a copy of updated care plans.

    For health promotion: This is a good time to raise the profile of long-term conditions (e.g. local media, open days). Patients can be given a pack to explain what they have to do, how they can get more information and how to get the best out of the health service.

For PAR: Two stakeholder workshops are useful in this season to finalise details of the improvement project(s) for that year. This is also a good time for leadership teams to attend a residential team-building workshop to plan the improvement projects.

August–October: season of concrete experience

For care: Actions in care plans can be reviewed alongside the flu campaign.

For health promotion: A rolling programme of health-promotion courses covers many topics.

For PAR: This season is a good time to undertake an evaluated improvement project.

November–December: season of reflection

For care, health promotion and PAR: This is a good time for a stakeholder workshop to review learning from care plans and improvement projects, and agree project(s) and general strategy for the coming year.

Examples of modules for a 'citizen' health promotion course:

- What is good mental health?
- Making the home a healthy environment
- Managing conflict and building relationships
- Co-creating a healthy community
- Evaluating complex interventions
- Food, exercise and nutrition
- Life planning
- Making the third age the best age
- Keeping the mind young
- Managing your long-term condition

Routinely gathered data can evaluate case studies of integrated care

Complex interventions like integrated care can be difficult to evaluate because the outcomes are diverse and many are long term. Routinely gathered data can help with this task and other data can also be gathered when needed. Data can be aligned to practices (adjusted for things like patient numbers), geographic clusters of practices (adjusted for things like unemployment), boroughs (adjusted for things like infrastructure) and even countries (adjusted for things like wealth).

 Stoddart, G., Gale, R., Peat, C. and McInnes, S. (2011) Using routinely gathered data to evaluate locally led service improvements, *London Journal of Primary Care*, 4: 1, 38–43, DOI:10.1080/17571472.2011.11493326

We can use data to assess the impact of integrated working on different types of health improvement, both short term and long term:

- Well-being – the extent to which individuals feel that they have an aliveness of spirit, are able to interact creatively with others and rise above adversity
- Citizenship – the extent to which people feel they belong to a caring community and are ready to contribute to improvements
- Capacity – the extent to which individuals are able to help themselves and mobilise assets to improve things for themselves and their communities
- Economics – the cost-effectiveness of care

Measures to consider in these categories are described in Chapter 11.

Aligning routinely gathered data to geographic localities helps to develop comparative case studies. Discussions between case-study sites helps to cross-pollinate ideas, as well as generate a healthy combination of competition and collaboration.

Real-time strategic change

Real-time strategic change is a form of *large group event* (Chapter 10) that is particularly suited to a health system. It involves facilitated debate between different leadership teams as though in a role play. But the people who are doing the roles are the people who genuinely hold those roles, so they are 'role playing' their real roles. In 'role' they challenge each other, yet remain appreciative and supportive in other ways. The sense of theatre allows people to hear difficult things with less defensiveness. After an encounter the various groups go away to rethink their positions, either within the same event or at a subsequent one. They lobby other groups and negotiate partnerships. Then they reconvene in a series of encounters that help everyone to adapt to everyone else. This process can continue for months and years, and can even become embedded as the routine way to operate.

A powerful application of real-time strategic change is to link it to a leadership course (Chapter 4). Practice, locality and system leadership teams become students who use their everyday work as material to learn how to lead. The course organisers also convene large group events that allow them to interact with purchasers, providers and other policy-making groups to learn and co-evolve, co-creating communities for health.

Exercise: identify relationship-building activities

Identify existing events and activities that stimulate creative conversations between different partners in your case study. Consider ways that they could connect for greater effect (e.g. by cascading ideas from one to another or a shared project).

Chapter 4

Infrastructure of facilitation and communication

Key message: An infrastructure of facilitation and communication can support cycles of learning and change for integrated care and collaborative health promotion.

In this chapter:

- 'Hard' and 'soft' ways of thinking need to be intertwined
- Integrating 'hard' and 'soft' ways of thinking is a life skill
- Applied research units can harness different kinds of authority and ways of thinking
- Learning sets for leadership teams can stimulate whole-system learning and change
- Live manuals and interactive bulletins keep people engaged
- Traditional, 'heroic' leaders are also needed
- Primary care needs strategic partners
- Things that strategic partners can do
- Exercise: engage strategic partners

'Hard' and 'soft' ways of thinking need to be intertwined

To successfully navigate complex things like community-oriented integrated care, people need to think in 'hard' and 'soft' ways at the same time. They need to define accurately what is known and sensitively explore what is not. They need to tightly uphold the law and be understanding of good reasons to break it. They need both mindsets at the same time.

The terms 'hard' and 'soft' come from systems theory. They refer to 'hard systems' that have clear boundaries and predictable, linear effects, and 'soft systems' that are interactive. The cardiovascular system is a hard system in the sense that blood flows in one predictable direction – like a machine. Exchange of nutrients across a cell membrane is a soft system in that different things happen depending on the nutrients being exchanged. They do not imply difficulty. Indeed the 'soft' activity of discerning the right thing to do in a complex situation is usually harder to do well than the 'hard' activity of precisely following a protocol.

Hard infrastructure for integrated working includes decision support and hospital admission avoidance schemes. Soft infrastructure includes mentorship, resilience and self-care. Hard outcomes include diseases cured. Soft outcomes include people feeling loved. Hard actions are purposeful – they do things to people. Soft actions are empowering – they help people to do things for themselves.

Hard activities are circumscribed. You can see them from a distance. They fit onto a bar graph. You can count and cost them. They are 'real' in the sense that you can touch them. Soft activities are more difficult to delineate. The spotlight cannot shine on them precisely because they are inter-relational. They are things like a culture of collaboration and people who listen and appreciate in ways that make others feel confident. Their empowering effects are felt more than seen; they are often only noticed when they are no longer there.

Combining hard and soft skills is the route to success in complex situations. The useful effect of combining them is obvious in teams where different people take *different* roles – for example the 'straight man' and 'funny man' in comedy and the 'good cop' and 'bad cop' in policing.

More difficult is to weave them together in *one* role.

Integrating 'hard' and 'soft' ways of thinking is a life skill

Chapter 15 explains that we combine 'hard' and 'soft' ways of thinking by linking them to evolving stories. In the moment, we decide what to do by listening thoughtfully to different kinds of thing and responding to the overall sense rather than to each specific aspect. This is not a linear process. We oscillate between big picture and focused detail, between long-term vision and short-term steps, between reaching out and contracting in. And we choose actions that help to move the whole story forwards. Only later do we find out if our actions were good ones – we find out when positive, coherent stories result. Or not.

We need to do this instinctively. When learning the skills it helps to oscillate between different ways of thinking and acting as purposeful exercises, but when the skills are mastered we do it without thinking.

These skills are not specific to leadership of health care. They are *life skills*, used by everyone to creatively interact with others and live life forwards with optimism. They require us to combine hard and soft ways of thinking. They include:

- **Be alive in the moment:** Diseases can challenge that sense of vitality, yet they can also be used creatively to enhance it. 'Hard' treatment of a disease needs to be complemented with 'soft' emotional intelligence.
- **Adventure in an uncertain world,** able to live life forwards with optimism, see whole stories as well as individual facts, inquire into complex situations, learn from experience, and use all of these to turn bad into good. 'Hard' journey plans need to be complemented with 'soft' street wisdom.
- **Be a team player,** able to dip in and out of different kinds of project, making timely and synchronous contributions that make wholes more than the sum of the parts. 'Hard' team tasks need to be complemented with 'soft' listening and intuitive support.
- **Be a life-long, life-wide learner,** able to learn from and with others, reflect, challenge myself and others, and change my own behaviours and ways of

thinking. 'Hard' facts need to be complemented with 'soft' self-reflection and co-adaptation.

* **Be resilient,** able to bend like a reed in the wind without breaking under pressure and remain centred when things are turbulent – surfing the waves of life. 'Hard' personal fitness needs to be complemented with 'soft' networks of support.

Each of these skills can be learned at every stage of life. Both children and adults need to learn them through everyday encounters and also through projects and family life. Implications for society as a whole are discussed in Chapter 20.

PAUSE: How do you develop your own skills as a team player who is alive in the moment and able to adventure in a complex world with optimism and resilience?

Applied research units can harness different kinds of authority and ways of thinking

Leadership teams for integrated care need 'soft', 'people skills' and 'hard' technical competence. *Applied research units* are needed to develop these teams, evaluate their activities and publish their work. Local authorities, public health, universities and others can strategically build networks of leadership teams that have broad reach and impact.

Applied research units can help to bring together three different kinds of authority and ways of thinking to enhance the work of the leadership teams.

1   **Organisational authority:** Individual organisations like general practices, schools and clubs have 'lists' or 'members'. They can develop these people as a 'family' of health-aware individuals skilled at collaboration and self-help. Leadership is often paternalistic to guide 'family members' towards healthy behaviours.
2   **Community authority:** Leadership teams within a community (e.g. a geographic area or a network) can engage organisations through annual cycles of collective reflection and coordinated action. Leadership is often multidisciplinary and helps different constituents to make sense of their place within broader systems.
3   **Individual authority:** Individual 'heroic' leaders envision integrated systems, relentlessly argue for this approach, pilot ways to achieve it and communicate this broad vision in ways that different groups can understand.

Learning sets for leadership teams can stimulate whole-system learning and change

Applied research units can lead, or commission, learning sets that energise and re-energise leadership teams for integrated working. The effect of these is often more profound when participants come from different kinds of team – e.g. practice leadership teams, locality leadership teams, system leadership teams. They can help each other to understand the constraints and potential of different parts of a system, and from this devise good strategy. Such learning sets use the notion of a *spiral curriculum* – participants learn the same things again and again at different levels of complexity.

These learning sets should:

a)   Provide a learning space within which participants cross-pollinate ideas and challenge each other, recognising that no one can do everything, and everyone needs to relate their focused work to bigger pictures.

b)   Introduce theories of integrated working, including: i) development as *complex co-adaptation*; ii) leadership as *sense-making*; iii) balancing control and harmony through *organisational learning*; iv) *multi-paradigm inquiry* to see more of a whole system.

c)   Introduce theories and language of life skills for health: i) *health* as being alive in the moment; ii) development as *adventure* into uncertainty; iii) *team players* as those who make the whole more than the sum of its parts; iv) life-long, life-wide, *inter-generational learning*; v) *Resilience* – remaining balanced in turbulent times.

d)   Support the evaluation of case studies and writing for publication.

e)   Use principles of real-time strategic change (Chapter 10) to engage policymakers and facilitate system-wide learning and change.

f)   Evaluate initiatives using multiple methods (Chapters 11 and 16) to reveal impact on well-being, citizenship, capacity and economics.

Live manuals and interactive bulletins keep people engaged

Live manuals are discussed in Chapter 8. They provide up-to-date information of what different disciplines are meant to do at different times of year for a specific condition or topic. Different teams update different sections. Each includes information about:

*   Patient care, including a three-tier system for shared care (Chapter 2)
*   Education and decision support for practitioners
*   Community participation for health promotion and self-help
*   Quality assurance and improvement projects

A *project leadership team*, supported by local health communities, coordinates the writing of a manual to be used by primary care teams, both for care and for health promotion. It is web based, so that different parts can be updated by different teams. *Practice leadership teams* update the parts that describe how their own practice manages the topic. *Locality leadership teams* describe local services and improvement projects. *System leadership teams* describes the bigger picture of morbidity, strategy, policy and mega-trends.

Interactive bulletins stimulate feedback and discussion that help to keep the manual alive.

Traditional, 'heroic' leaders are also needed

The emphasis in this book is on networks of leadership teams because this has historically been neglected. More traditional individual leaders are still needed, and indeed members of leadership teams act as individual leaders much of the time.

Individual leaders are often developed through diplomas, masters and doctorates. They are often appointed to leadership roles within organisations. To create a synchrony of effort it is important that their leadership roles link with existing local infrastructure, including the applied research unit that develops local leadership teams.

Primary care needs strategic partners

There are many things that primary care cannot do alone. For example, here are four things for which local health communities need strategic partners.

Mental health

General practices, public health and local health communities need to serve 100 per cent of the population for health promotion, 10 per cent of the population that suffer transient anxiety and depression, and 1 per cent of the population who need more complex services and long-term support. They need to work with a variety of mental health services to do this.

Social factors contribute powerfully to mental illness and also to positive mental health, so local health communities also need to work with those who help people to develop good social support, skilled parenting and personal resilience, including social services, schools, faith groups and voluntary groups.

Long-term conditions

The rapidly increasing numbers of long-term conditions means that general practices and local health communities need to work with specialist practitioners and others to support shared care. An example is the three-tier model of shared care for diabetes described in Chapter 2. They need to work with academic colleagues to evaluate these models and with policymakers to apply the lessons to shared care for other long-term conditions.

Workforce training

New roles need to be developed all the time, so local health communities need to work with universities and colleges to explore how to best do this.

Research and publications

Local health communities need academic partners to research and evaluate service improvements, using multi-method, multi-perspective participatory action research. They need to be fluent at describing what happens in community-oriented integrated care.

Things that strategic partners can do

Coalitions of clinical commissioning groups, GP federations, local authorities, health and well-being boards, leaders of learning sets and shared leadership teams need to negotiate agreements with strategic partners to help develop health networks and local health communities. Here are some things that different strategic partners might be able to do.

- **Hospitals** can design and evaluate shared care for long-term conditions. They can provide educational support for generalists, including electronic and telephone advice.
- **Universities** can place students and evaluate service improvements. The students can go back to the same places year after year to see how things change over time.
- **Applied research units** can resource whole-system improvement projects, shared learning and leadership development.
- **Professional bodies** can provide vision for multidisciplinary team-working, global health and public health/primary care partnerships.
- **Out-of-hours services** can enhance daytime efforts with opportunistic input.
- **Public health and local authorities** can support a locality-based approach to health promotion, social care and evaluation.
- **Schools** can teach life skills for an integrated world. They can collaborate for primary care and public health for health promotion and parenting, feeding back information to primary care about service gaps and emerging need.
- **Voluntary groups** can help communities to help themselves.
- **Private companies** can provide funds and work placements. This could change the definition of 'public service ethos' away from its funding source (i.e. public or private) towards a commitment to work collaboratively for the health of whole populations.
- **Educational institutions** can provide leadership and resources for specific purposes (e.g. nurse training), for the dissemination of learning from case studies, and for conferences, leadership development and writing for publication.
- **Political parties** can use annual cycles of collaborative learning and coordinated change to develop local participatory democracy that identifies local health issues and supports local people to improve them.

Rather than engage solely at times of their interest, strategic partners should engage for at least three consecutive cycles. This helps to demonstrate their commitment to develop a community with long-term goals rather than short-term reactivity. It signals their commitment to the whole system rather than merely their own interests. Three cycles gives time to develop trusted relationships and to learn to value the collaborative processes.

Exercise: engage strategic partners

Consider organisational partner(s) in your case study who could help move forward your plans for development. Design a pilot project with them.

Part II

Integrating care and promoting health from local organisations

In Part II:

Who might find Part II useful?

This part is written primarily for leaders of community-based organisations that contribute to health and care, especially general practices, but also schools, pharmacists, voluntary groups and others. It describes how to lead integrating activities from small, semi-independent organisations. The small size means having to negotiate with fewer people, so leaders can often act quickly.

Leadership from a small, tight team has advantages. But it only works within its domains of authority and it can exclude people whose insights would lead to better strategy. It is also easy to leave out of the planning people from inside the organisation who are needed to keep everyone together, causing instability. The approach described in this part aims to avoid these disadvantages by setting leadership activities within a broader framework of whole-organisation learning and change.

Annual cycles of learning and change within the organisation are set within *seasons of care, health promotion and improvement* to make it easier to align the activities inside and outside the organisation. *Practice leadership teams* and *project leadership teams* work with *locality leadership teams* and *system leadership teams* to integrate each other's effects. *Live manuals* remind different people what they need to do at different times of year. *Large group events* help people to creatively interact.

The image to support this section: Interactive juggling

Integrated care is too complex to control directly. There are too many things to do, and to know. Also, control on its own stifles innovation. It prevents people from thinking for themselves. The system has to help people from different parts to interact with others creatively, so their combined effort is more than the sum of the parts. This is helped when individual practitioners are skilled at juggling many things. Networks of 'jugglers' can integrate activities across different organisational boundaries.

At the highest level jugglers do it 'blind' – they instinctively know where to throw things, and others know how to catch what they throw. This kind of success comes from years of practice and networks of high-performing teams. It develops best with supportive infrastructure and facilitative leadership.

Primary care practitioners need to know where other 'jugglers' are, so that they can refer patients appropriately, seek advice and establish shared care. They need to practise their interactions, to be mutually supportive and creative.

Leadership teams from different organisations need to work together. Together these 'jugglers' can see things that should be improved in all parts of a system. They are well placed to pilot new ways of working.

Introduction to Part II: primary care is a good place to lead integrated care

Primary care is a good place to lead integrated care. The closer you get to where people live their everyday lives the more you can see the many factors that impact on their health and illnesses, and the need for coordinated actions to address them. Away from the local area, for example hospitals, conversations revolve around more focused concerns, and so naturally lead to more focused actions.

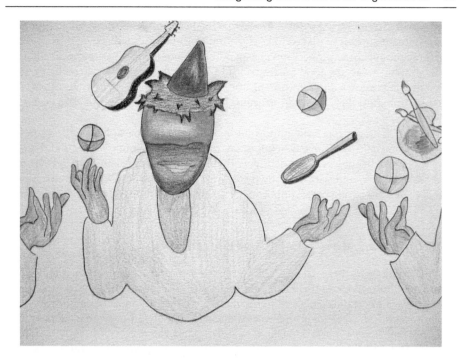

Figure II Interactive juggling

Primary care has good raw ingredients. It has highly motivated, intelligent practitioners and managers who every day encounter the complexities of health and the idiosyncrasies of people. In addition, the range of tasks makes multi-disciplinary team-working inevitable. General practitioners (GPs) work with nurse practitioners and practice nurses in *practice teams*. Community-based doctors, nurses and multiple therapists work in *extended primary care teams*. Specialists and generalists work in *long-term condition teams*.

Generalists are key to integration because they cover everything. People present to specialists to answer a problem that relates to that speciality. During a consultation, no one is likely to ask an eye surgeon to sort out a knee problem or control their diabetes. What this means is that the specialist expectation of integrated care is to identify and solve problems one at a time. Specialists expect integrated care to help patients to 'step up' to and 'step down' from their speciality.

In contrast, people present to generalists with multiple intertwined problems. Some are immediate short-term problems, but often more important problems lurk below the surface. Patients have long-term conditions that require monitoring. They have chronic dis-eases that gnaw away like a constant headache – relationship difficulties, dissatisfaction at work, stress, loss of purpose. This means that the generalist expectation of integrated care is to enable various practitioners to share care for patients with complex conditions, and to access resources that help people to help themselves.

The reason why primary care is a good place to lead integrated care goes beyond the nature of primary care consultations. Primary care practitioners work regularly with practitioners from every part of the system – medical, surgical, social, mental health. So they are uniquely well placed to see how multiple dis-eases interact within a person and how multiple practitioners interact within a system – and how to improve both.

Geographic areas are good places to lead integrated working because the geographic boundary allows different organisations to lead different aspects, and from this build a community for care and for health improvements. This approach is discussed in Part III.

But general practice has one important ingredient that geographic localities do not have – *the practice list*. Similarly, schools, pharmacists and voluntary groups and others have lists of 'stakeholders' who identify with them. Local organisations can work with their stakeholders, and with their own staff, to develop them as a network or family that is skilled at sharing care, supporting self-help and leading improvement projects.

Bromley by Bow Health Partnership

The Bromley by Bow Centre (BBBC) started in 1984, initially as a church initiative to regenerate the local community – one of the most deprived areas in the UK. They established a children's nursery, a dance school, a community cafe and a series of art studios and workshops and became a force for local health improvement.

In 1997 the Bromley by Bow Centre Healthy Living Centre (general practice) was opened, creating a partnership between general practice and BBBC for health and care. This allowed a combination of traditional medical care with the development of a local community for health with a social enterprise arm.

The practice now has three surgeries and a walk-in centre, working with around 27,000 patients. Bromley-by-Bow remains a deprived area – half of the Centre's patients can't read or write and a third of consultations are conducted in a language other than English.

The practice uses a philosophy of co-design, including people from the local area, and various partner organisations. The doctor/patient relationship is seen as one that encourages self-care, equality and empowerment. During consultations, GPs sit side by side with their patients, so they can look at the computer screen together if necessary.

The practice signposts a range of local initiatives to help people to help themselves, both on its website and on its waiting-room walls. For example, it advertises courses that teach how to run a business, and self-help for chronic conditions. It hosts a number of community-focused initiatives, for example Citizen's Advice Bureau and 'Chatter/Natter'.

Their website describes ways to think about illness as well as health. The practice wants patients to be experts in their own health, so they guide patients to self-care and online help as well as encourage involvement in developing the practice.

 Bromley by Bow Health Partnership www.bbbhp.co.uk/

Chapter 5

Annual cycles of participatory action research

Key message: Annual cycles of collaborative inquiry and coordinated change support continuous quality improvements and integrated working. They can be led by locally based, semi-independent organisations such as general practices, pharmacies and schools.

In this chapter:

- Set participatory action research within seasons of learning and change
- An annual timeline for participatory action research
- Engage strategic partners in cycles of participatory action research
- Start where you can, and have realistic goals
- What a practice leadership team does in seasons of care and improvement
- Draft letter to patients with diabetes about shared care
- Three consulting styles for medical matters
- Three consulting concerns for integrated care
- Four domains of evaluation
- Exercise: devise an annual cycle of activity

Set participatory action research within seasons of learning and change

Primary care practitioners are great 'doers'. They are good at getting their individual jobs done. They are less used to working within teams, organisations and systems. Reflection and learning are mainly considered to be solitary activities. A good way to get everyone to be better team players within the whole organisation is to wrap annual activities up into collaborative inquiries. This means that at different times of the year people from the organisation stand back and review where things are going in the light of the journey so far; then they get their heads down again to do their work in slightly different ways. In the organisational development literature this is called 'freeze–unfreeze'. An approach that helps to do this is called *participatory action research* (PAR) (see also Chapter 11).

Chapter 3 describes four 'seasons of learning and change' when practitioners from different organisations and backgrounds naturally do similar things at the same time. PAR can be set onto these seasons, providing a way to build relationships within an organisation, network or community, and integrate different efforts for care and health improvements. PAR can be led from geographic areas (Part III), or from a single organisation (this part).

PAR gets people to contribute to (participatory) an inquiry (research) and do something positive about what they find (action). For example, they might use data about illnesses to inform health improvements. Participation stimulates a broad sense of ownership that helps to sustain improvements and motivates people to take part in future.

Like *experienced-based co-design* (Chapter 11), PAR punctuates periods of activity with events where stakeholders stand back to reflect on the emerging data and their daily experience. The *research community* adjusts the direction according to what it has learned.

It takes at least three cycles of PAR for people to trust it, so plan them at the outset. The first cycle usually feels a bit chaotic and participants are surprised when it achieves anything valuable. When the second cycle also succeeds, participants really start to see its value. When the third cycle again succeeds many people become advocates instead of sceptics. The really powerful effects come when the cycles of research and development become embedded as the routine way to operate – as annual cycles of inquiry, learning and change.

You can lead a PAR project from a single organisation, such as a general practice, but it will be more effective when it complements other local improvement projects (Part III). People often use PAR when they have a large transformation project to undertake – the scale of change makes it obvious that broad ownership is needed. But you can use the processes in more modest projects too, helping people to learn the processes in a less exposed way.

An annual timeline for participatory action research

The timeline below describes stages of a participatory action research project led by a single organisation such as a general practice, set within the seasons of learning and change described in Chapter 3.

An idea emerges (scrutinised at a workshop in November/ December)

a) **Choose an aspect** of care that you want to improve. Let's take mental health or diabetes. It might be an improvement within your practice (e.g. set up a practice diabetes clinic). It might be a locality improvement (e.g. pilot mental health support workers). Or it might be a whole system improvement (e.g. pilot a three -tier system of shared care for mental health as described in Chapter 2). Better to start small.

b) **Convene a multidisciplinary practice leadership team:** It should include people who have different insights into the topic. Agree with them the rationale for the project, including what is lacking in the present situation and the long-term vision.

c) **Define a research question(s)** that helps everyone to puzzle over the question being asked in the project. Examples of questions are:

- 'What should happen in our proposed diabetes clinic?'
- 'What should mental health support workers do?'
- 'What are the obstacles to setting up a three-tier system of diabetes care?'

- 'How can we best help patients with intermittent acute mental illness?'
- 'How can we promote good parenting skills in new parents?'

Bring the relevant system into view (January–March)

d) **List the stakeholders** relevant to your question. You can list people whose support or insights are useful and those whose behaviour might need to change as a result of the project (e.g. practice staff, patients, community nurses, allied health professionals, specialists, commissioners, managers, academics).

e) **Draw a diagram** of how the people in the 'whole system' connect now (see 'case study' in the Introduction), and a second diagram to show how they are expected to connect in the new system you are planning.

f) **Undertake rapid appraisal and backwards mapping** exercises (Chapter 7) to deepen your understanding of the issues. Then write a project plan and get colleagues to critique it.

Second Stakeholder Workshop (April) agrees the general vision and rules of engagement

g) **Facilitate a stakeholder workshop:** You can use an established format (Chapter 10) or design your own (Chapter 8). Get participants to critique and agree:

- The research question(s)
- Changes that might be piloted
- Data to evaluate progress
- Key contacts from each organisation
- An oversight team
- Shared leadership teams
- Links with similar initiatives

Set up project systems

h) **The project leadership team(s):**

- Meets regularly (e.g. weekly) to plan the project
- Gathers data
- Writes a regular (e.g. monthly) interactive bulletin to practice staff and significant others to describe progress
- Prepares project materials, including timelines, literature, project plan, evaluation
- Creates links with similar teams from other places to cross-pollinate ideas

Third stakeholder workshop (July) agrees the specific project

i) **Facilitate a third workshop** at which participants agree:

- Question(s) to be answered
- Changes to be piloted

- Data to be gathered
- Roles in the project

Undertake the project (September–November)

j)   Make the pilot changes and gather data

Fourth stakeholder workshop (November/December) makes sense of data in the light of the experiences of participants

k)   **Facilitate a fourth workshop** to review progress, conclude implications for policy, agree a focus for the next year's improvement project, and agree a team(s) to lead it.

l)   **Re-draw the diagram** of how the people should connect in the envisioned new system. Identify data to be routinely generated to check that the changes are sustained.

Start a new PAR cycle

m) **The new leadership team(s)**, with a new research question, starts the whole sequence again (December) and brings a new system into view (January–March)

n)   **Organise training events** (January–March), for others to learn from the work done in the previous cycle and critique the plans of the work that has just started.

You can do this solely with people from your organisation, but it will be more powerful if you include people from different parts of the relevant system and link with their initiatives.

Engage strategic partners in cycles of participatory action research

The seasons are called planning, coordinated actions, concrete experience and reflection. They are the four stages of Kolb's learning cycle: abstract conceptualisation–active experimentation–concrete experience–reflective observation (Chapter 19).

Kolb reminds us that people learn and change by reflecting ideas (theory, hunches, prejudices) against their lived experience, then trying new things out and reflecting again. Organisations, systems and communities learn in the same way, when the members move from ideas to experiments to experience to observations to ideas to experiments. The four seasons frame cycles of organisational learning and change.

Strategic partners can align their work to the cycles of participatory action research:

- Public health, local authorities, voluntary groups and schools can align their plans for horizontal integration for health promotion and community development.
- Hospitals can align their plans for vertical integration for care pathway evaluation, leadership development, information about services, patient packs.
- Universities can align student placements, funding applications, training and research.

Strategic partners can also help to make primary care waiting rooms places where people can learn about other opportunities – a 'one stop shop' for self-help and community action.

Start where you can, and have realistic goals

There is no perfect place to start annual cycles of participatory action research. Start wherever you can. Don't let the long list of tasks above worry you – they are things you would do anyway, set out in a timeline. Listing them like this allows you to do each quickly, with confidence, rather than constantly having to reinvent the plan. Remember:

1 Avoid overly ambitious aims that can cause people unnecessary stress. It is better to have modest aims that participants can easily achieve and enjoy.
2 You will need to remind people of the processes they are engaged in. People are used to short-term tasks and will easily forget that they are on a long-term journey.

What a practice leadership team does in seasons of care and improvement

Here are things that a practice leadership team might do to improve diabetes care:

January–March: planning

The shared leadership team engages patients and strategic partners to co-design service improvements and care-plan updates, applying learning from the previous year. They undertake a rapid appraisal (Chapter 7) to better understand the issues and pilot materials.

April–July: coordinated actions

In April, the team invites all patients with diabetes to collect their forms (for blood and urine tests and retinal checks) and a pack containing home monitoring advice (e.g. blood glucose and blood pressure) and other useful information. Each patient is sent a (text) message with their results for HbA1C, fasting blood glucose, cholesterol and urinary albumin/creatinine ratio to record in their home record. Patients book an appointment to discuss the results.

A GP, nurse and health care assistant holds daily or weekly *annual care plan update clinics* (half-hour appointments). They work in adjacent consulting rooms so that they can dip in and out of each other's consultations. Tests are reviewed and goals for the year negotiated. Patients are asked to agree to provide data from home monitoring at agreed times. A review date is agreed to coincide with their autumn flu jab.

All the shared leadership teams prepare to contribute to locality whole-system events (Chapters 8 and 10) in April and July. Plans for improving the diabetes system for that year can be agreed at these events.

August–October: concrete experience

Those who have not updated their care plan are chased up.

Regular *diabetes (or long-term condition) review clinics* help patients to achieve their goals (15-minute appointments). GPs, nurses and health care assistants consult in adjacent rooms as before. The flu vaccination is given.

A rolling programme of health-promotion courses takes place.

The improvement project is completed, gathering qualitative and quantitative *outcome and improvement measures* (Chapter 11).

November–December: reflection

The practice leadership team holds a stakeholder event (Chapters 8 and 10) at which people with different perspectives review progress with the practice improvement projects, agree plans for the coming year, reform the shared leadership teams and start the next cycle. This can be done in collaboration with other practices and strategic partners.

Draft letter to patients with diabetes about shared care

We are writing to let you know about our system for caring for your diabetes.

Most of the time you will be seen in the practice diabetes clinic [days/times of the clinics].

From time to time you may also go elsewhere for health-promotion courses, for dietician advice, and for eye and feet screening. The practice will work closely with local specialists to make sure that you receive the best care.

Between April and August we will update your Care Plan. It will include your own targets for the year ahead.

Please collect your forms for the Annual Tests (blood and urine) from reception (from 1 April), and get the tests done. We will send you a text message of your results. When you have received this, get an appointment for your annual care plan update.

You will find a pack waiting for you at reception. It contains:

- How the system works – what needs to be done when and where
- How to do your own home monitoring – e.g. blood sugar, blood pressure. Suggestions for things you may like to include in your care plan
- Useful agencies and courses

When your care plan has been updated, we will send a copy to the out-of-hours service. This means that if you ever need to contact them when the surgery is closed they will have some information about you.

We need your permission to share your information with them, so please sign the enclosed copy of this letter and return it to us.

Signed: Care Plan Coordinator   Named GP
P.S. Your forms will be available at reception from 1 April

Three consulting styles for medical matters

General practitioners need to switch effortlessly between three consulting styles, of which one is the structured approach to care plans described above. The others are reactive care (patients presenting with problems) and emergency care (things have to be done in a hurry).

The three consulting styles require different approaches and different resources:

1   **Reactive care:** Works thoughtfully from the presenting complaint, using a 'narrative-based' style of consulting (Chapter 14). This style allows issues that might impact on health to surface (e.g. other diseases, emotional and social issues, their care plan).
2   **Planned care:** This follows the care-plan goals, using protocols and patient data.
3   **Emergency care:** This style solves an immediate threat, e.g. stroke, appendicitis, acute mental illness, child abuse.

Reactive care needs a combination of booked and unbooked consultations. Planned care needs patient packs to explain what they have to do themselves and by when. Emergency care needs a clinical room with a full range of emergency equipment.

Three consulting concerns for integrated care

In all consulting styles (reactive, planned care and emergency care), practitioners need to combine three aims of consultations:

1   *Treat diseases:* Everything to do with addressing specific problems, whether overt or hidden, medical or non-medical, including long-term conditions, and mental, physical, social and spiritual concerns.
2   *Promote health:* Everything to do with helping someone to feel whole and vital, able to reach out to others, rise above adversity and take control of their life.
3   *Improve systems:* Everything to do with improving systems of care within and beyond the consulting room.

Launer's approach to consulting helps to move between these different aims. He calls it 'narrative-based primary care' (Chapter 14). It is a form of active listening that follows the 'asides' made by a patient as though an everyday conversation. It helps a clinician and a patient to consider many different things at the same time and weave them together to make a positive story. This approach also helps to develop a care plan that considers non-medical aspects as well as medical.

Four domains of evaluation

General practices need to evaluate the impact of their various activities on a range of outcomes, beyond treating illnesses. One question is what these outcomes might be?

In 2015 the *Connected Communities Project* was published by the Royal Society of Arts and its partners at the University of Central Lancashire (UCLan) and the London

School of Economics (LSE). They identified four different kinds of outcome from interventions designed to build communities. They are:

1   **A wellbeing dividend.** Social connectedness correlates strongly with wellbeing.
2   **A citizenship dividend.** Latent power within local communities can be activated.
3   **A capacity dividend.** Networks and relationships positively affect everyone.
4   **An economic dividend.** Social relationships improve employability and health, and create health and welfare savings.

 Report: Community Capital – The value of connected communities. 28 October 2015. www.thersa.org/discover/publications-and-articles/reports/community-capital-the-value-of-connected-communities/

These categories help to identify data that practices might want to routinely generate to evaluate the overall effect of the practice:

a)   **Well-being:** Care plans updated. Change in tracer markers (e.g. blood-sugar control)
b)   **Citizenship:** Self-care. Participation in improvement projects. Use of services by patients who have and don't have a care plan
c)   **Capacity:** Patient and staff satisfaction and competence. Number of leadership teams and stakeholder feedback of their effectiveness
d)   **Economic:** Unscheduled consultations and admissions of patients with and without a care plan

In addition to evaluating individual practice performance, the effect of clusters of practices (Part III) can be evaluated in a similar way. Many public service organisations, including general practices and hospitals, routinely code clinical episodes. Data can be amalgamated from these databases to gain insights into the impact of complex interventions by practice, locality or borough.

Exercise: devise an annual cycle of activity

Develop an annual timetable of activity. Use *participatory action research* to lead a pilot project(s). Consider what routinely gathered data could contribute to evaluation of the project(s).

Chapter 6

Live manuals

Key message: When practitioners and managers from different parts of the system help to generate an information resource, the sense of ownership gained means that they are more likely to use the resource wisely.

In this chapter:

- Live manuals help to build teams
- Internal and external leadership teams both contribute to live manuals
- Work programmes that might benefit from live manuals
- Amalgamating and dividing manuals
- Getting started with live manuals
- Structure and content of a live manual
- Keeping a live manual alive
- Example: live manual for child safeguarding
- Example: live manual for diabetes
- Example: live manual for mental health
- Exercise: write a live manual

Live manuals help to build teams

The previous chapter showed how practice leadership teams can engage people inside and outside the practice in annual cycles of collaborative inquiry and coordinated improvements, and evaluate their combined impact. This chapter shows how *live manuals* help everyone to remember what they have to do in these cycles.

At first sight a live manual looks like any other policy document – it describes leaders of work programmes, care pathways, protocols, audits and training. The main differences are that it is web-based, continually updated and, crucially, used every day as a live, useful resource. Different teams are responsible for updating different parts.

Different live manuals for the same practice can complement each other. Each describes the local context, principles of operation, timetables of events, key contacts and strategic partners. They describe long-term outcomes as well as short-term goals. They help to describe the practice and its related organisations as a *case study* and can include data to show how it compares with others (Chapter 11).

Live manuals also help everyone to value the contributions of the large number of people in different parts of the system. Individual practitioners can have only marginal influence on the overall health of their local population. A live manual shows how different interventions can enhance each other with powerful collective impact.

The process of creating and maintaining a live manual can build trust, motivate people to collaborate and generate new ideas. Using and revising the manual provides the opportunity to revitalise that trust, and consider new ideas about how to improve health.

PAUSE: How do you remind people of how the practice systems work?

Internal and external leadership teams both contribute to live manuals

Writing and updating a live manual helps practice leadership teams to develop their professional networks and their knowledge of the topic at the same time. By putting the plans into action and auditing them, they also improve team-working.

Differences between a live manual and a traditional protocol are:

- Teams from different disciplines write and maintain it, overseen by a multidisciplinary leadership team from those disciplines (or organisations).
- Practice leadership teams work with their counterparts in local practices and the broader system to align the content of different manuals.
- Different manuals have a similar structure to make them feel familiar.
- Manuals go beyond tasks to also explain education, community development and improvement projects.
- Live manuals are used every day for a variety of purposes. They actually support people as they work.

Work programmes that might benefit from live manuals

Live manuals can be useful for many different general practice (organisational) purposes. Here are some suggestions.

Strategic planning teams
- Strategy and projects, including overview of the work of all teams
- Finance and staffing
- Patient engagement and quality improvement
- Governance – e.g. complaints, compliments, significant events, monitoring projects
- Staff development – e.g. clinical updating, leadership skills

Clinical teams
- Surgeries – day-to-day organisation
- Care plans – personal teams for individual patients
- Safeguarding registers – personal teams for those on safeguarding registers
- Locum pack
- Overview of how to think in different clinical situations

Care pathway teams

- Diabetes, heart, lung, cancer
- End-of-life care
- Safeguarding (children and adults)
- Mental health and mental illness
- Women's health, cervical smears and family planning
- Child health and childhood immunisations
- Clinics – minor surgery, long-term conditions, anticoagulation, etc.

Data management teams

- Internal communication – e.g. tasks, telephones and meetings
- External communication – e.g. out-of-hours contacts, letters, results
- Audit – monitoring, targets, reports, e.g. non-elective admissions and out-of-hours contacts, referrals, quality outcomes framework, care plans
- Information technology support

Seasons of care teams

- Annual cycle of care-plan activity
- Patient communication – e.g. care-plan update, flu vaccinations, health promotion
- Patient-held care plans and updates for out-of-hours services
- Patient access to records

Communication teams

- Internal communication
- External communication
- Huddle – five-minute (standing) review of the day's work

Amalgamating and dividing manuals

In some practices a few individuals will be in most teams. In others, broader participation will be helpful. Use the writing and updating of them strategically to develop leadership teams, a sense of ownership of the organisational strategy and a culture of team-learning.

As far as possible keep the structure of different manuals the same, to make them more familiar to the reader and to allow several to be updated at the same time.

If you combine manuals (e.g. for heart and lung care) keep the original titles at the top so they can remain linked to the manuals of other practices. Also, combine them in ways that suit the configuration of your local health-care system. For example, if the heart and kidney services are in one hospital and lung and cancer services in another, combine your manuals accordingly. Even better, write the manuals with them.

You may need to expand or divide some programmess to fit your local situation. For example, 'safeguarding children' might be separated into 'children with special needs' and 'families at risk'. Mental illness might be separated into *severe enduring mental illness, cognitive impairment, anxiety and depression* and *acute psychosis*. In different places these separate programmes will be led by different teams, and you can align the manuals to those teams.

Getting started with live manuals

A live manual might start as a short document with a list of headings to be built on later. The team that oversees it identifies when the time is right to write the sections. The live manual could be developed to link with a participatory action research project (Chapter 5), or as a collaboration with others. You can use the writing of a live manual to build teams:

- A *practice leadership team* can meet regularly to write and update the practice manual. This is a good way to develop the practice as a learning organisation.
- A *locality leadership team* can coordinate the writing of different manuals, led by different practices. This is a good way to build a local community for health.
- A *system leadership team* can work with multiple organisations across a borough or coalition of boroughs to support an aligned approach. This approach is particularly good at building a network of leadership teams for whole system improvements.

Structure and content of a live manual

A live manual needs to be written so the reader can quickly get the information they need. It is written for a general reader. Rather than try to say everything it should link to more detailed guidance for the few who might need it (e.g. prescribing insulin).

To aid familiarity it needs a structure that can be adapted to other programmes and updated by different teams. For example:

a) **The system of care** (key contacts, practice procedures, care pathways)
b) **Education** (training and decision support)
c) **Community participation** (self-help, health promotion)
d) **Quality improvement** (local health community meetings, improvement projects)

Keeping a live manual alive

A live manual has to be up to date. *System leadership teams* can update the sections that describe whole systems of care and education, whereas sections that describe local initiatives are best updated by practice and locality leadership teams.

Updated by system leadership teams, working with practice leadership teams

a) **The system of care:** Key contacts inside and outside the practice. Roles of team members, intermediate care and hospital care. Seasons of care. Care pathways.
b) **Education:** Training courses for practitioners. Decision support – electronic, telephone and e-mail. Communication and external data.

Updated by locality leadership teams, working with practice leadership teams

c)   **Community participation:** Training courses for patients. Self help and advice lines. Timetable of health promotion, patient participation and community development.

d)   **Quality Improvement:** Local health community improvement projects, timeline of annual activity. Evaluation measures (well-being, citizenship, capacity, economic).

Example: live manual for child safeguarding

a) The system of care

1   Practice leads for the child safeguarding programme
2   Emergency contacts
3   What to do if you suspect abuse
4   Missing children
5   Brief overview of management of child abuse (pointing to other resources for those who require more detail)

b) Education

6   Definitions
7   Things that might indicate child abuse, or need for better parenting
8   Promoting good child health and parenting in daily practice
9   Decision support and training
10 Resources

c) Community participation

11 Health Promotion – self-help groups, parenting classes and videos, campaigns
12 Community development initiatives

d) Continuous quality improvement

13 This year's improvement projects
14 Timetable of activity for collaborative improvement
15 Monitoring and quality assurance
16 Appendices

Example: live manual for diabetes

a) The system of care

1   Practice leads for diabetes care
2   Practice system of diabetes care including home monitoring and care plans
3   Care pathway – community and hospital care contacts and clinics (tiers two and three)

4   Criteria for diabetes diagnosis and targets for control
5   DVLA (driving) recommendation
6   Brief overview of diabetes management (pointing to other resources for specific clinical guidance and patient information)

b) Education

7   Definitions of IDDM and NIDDM (insulin and non-insulin dependent diabetes mellitus). Statistics of prevalence and service use
8   When to consider diabetes
9   Lifestyle to prevent and manage diabetes
10 Decision support and training options
11 Other resources

c) Community participation

12 Health Promotion – self-help groups, 'Understand your diabetes' course, campaigns
13 Local research projects

d) Continuous quality improvement

14 This year's improvement projects
15 Timetable of activity for collaborative improvement
16 Monitoring and quality assurance
17 Appendices

Example: live manual for mental health

a) The system of care

1   Care pathway – clinics and contacts and clinics (tiers one, two and three)
2   Decision support and training options
3   DVLA (driving) recommendation
4   Links to patient information
5   Brief overview of mental illness management (pointing to other resources for those who need more specific clinical guidance)

b) Education

6   Understanding **mental health** (narrative unity, resilience, well-being, living life forwards)
7   Understanding **mental illness** (fragmentation of the self, illness categories, treatments)
8   Mental illness and mental health throughout a life (life course, parenting, community)
9   Things general practice can do (sequence of consultations, PHQ9, GAD7, red flags)

10 Things patients/families can do (reflective diaries, exercise, environments for health)
11 Lifestyle that promotes good mental health and controls mental illness
12 Other resources

c) Community participation

13 Health promotion – self-help groups, understanding good mental health course and videos, campaigns
14 Research projects

d) Continuous quality improvement

15 This year's improvement project
16 Timetable of activity for collaborative improvement
17 Monitoring and Quality Assurance
18 Appendices

Exercise: write a live manual

Consider which topics in your case study would most benefit from a live manual. Who will write it? Ask them to make a start.

Chapter 7

How to see connections between parts and wholes

Key message: Leaders of community-oriented integrated care need images, theories and methods that help them to think clearly in complex situations.

In this chapter:

- We need to continually move between different ways of thinking and looking
- Images that reveal connections between actions and co-evolving wholes

    o A human body
    o A garden
    o Sailing at sea
    o Music, dance and the performing arts

- Theories that help to engage with complexity

    o Leadership as sense-making
    o Health as positive narrative unity
    o Evolution as a complex co-adaptation
    o Relationships as a co-constructed sense of 'we'

- Methods that inform good decisions in complex situations

    o Rapid appraisal
    o Backwards mapping
    o Systems mapping
    o Action learning

- Exercise: use techniques that see parts and wholes

We need to continually move between different ways of thinking and looking

To see the health of someone as well as their diseases, it helps to think of every situation as a story-in-evolution. Facts are like still photograph of a feature film – useful, but they do not say it all. You need to move continually between focused detail and 'bigger pictures'. You need to see steps *and* journeys *and* destinations. This chapter includes images, theories and methods that will help you to do this.

If you spend too much time thinking about bigger pictures you will lose a sense of being grounded. Spend too much time thinking about detail and you will lose a sense of meaning. Spend too much time thinking about interconnections and you will lose a sense of yourself. Thinking of it all at the same time can frazzle your brain.

In order to remain balanced, you need to move continually between these different ways of thinking and looking at the world. Helpful images, theories and methods show how individual parts and emerging wholes make sense together. They help to make leaps of intuition.

Take the example of walking in a wood. If you want to adventure within it, rather than merely keep to the established routes, you will be helped by *images* of the whole wood and its paths (e.g. a map), *theories* of what happens in different parts of the wood (e.g. which berries are safe to eat), and *methods* to assess dangers and opportunities (e.g. binoculars).

Images that reveal connections between actions and co-evolving wholes

Gareth Morgan explains how to use images and metaphors to see movement from the past into the future. Different images lead to different understandings of how the world behaves, and lead to different actions. He examines what happens when we think of organisations as *machines, organisms, brains, culture, political systems, psychic prisons, flux and transformation and instrument of domination*. Each image has strengths and limitations.

 Morgan G. *Images of Organization*. Sage: Thousand Oaks, CA, 1997

Morgan describes how different images see some things and not others:

> When we say 'the man is a lion' we use the image of a lion to draw attention to the lion-like aspects of the man. The metaphor frames our understanding of the man in a distinctive yet partial way . . . thus, in drawing attention to the lion-like bravery, strength or ferocity of the man, the metaphor glosses over the fact that the same person may well also be a pig, a devil, a saint, a bore, or a recluse.
>
> (p. 4)

To get the right balance between treating illness and promoting health, integrated care needs images that simultaneously reveal its machine-like aspects and its living systems-like aspects. They need to reveal functional activities (that need to be done in a precise, machine-like, prescribed way) and emergent activities (that open out creative opportunities). Here are four images that help to do this:

- Human body
- A garden
- Sailing at sea
- Music, dance and the performing arts

Image – human body

The basic unit of life is not a particle but a cell. It is a living system, alive with creative potential that reaches out to 'play' with other cells. The creative interactions result in mutual co-adaptation that forms larger organs. Networks of organs become integrated to make a whole body, bound together by the trillions of 'trusted relationships' that were developed during their co-creation – each plays its agreed part. Nerves and a variety of messenger hormones provide feedback and control that retain harmony throughout the whole body.

These multi-communicating 'soft systems' aspects of a human body are not the whole picture. A human body also has machine-like features. For example, the cardiovascular system. This is a 'hard system' – blood flows in one, predictable direction. Similarly the nervous system, the lymphatic system, gastrointestinal system, and so on.

Cells in a human body conform to 'ground rules'. These are mutually agreed arrangements developed during their creation. Breaking them threatens the integrity of the whole. Failure of heart muscles to pump in the expected way causes heart failure, just as cars that fail to drive on the agreed side of a road cause accidents. Cells that aggressively attack others are called cancers, and people that do this are called terrorists. Blocked arteries cause limbs to whither just as blocked minds prevent understanding.

Implications of the image of a human body

The image of a human body helps us to see both machine-like and living system-like aspects of integrated care and human relationships. Individual organisations such as general practices and clusters of practices can be nurtured as cells within the 'body' of health care, just as two people can work together to develop a trusted relationship. Leadership teams span different 'organs', or organ(isation)s, to facilitate co-evolution of the whole system.

Image – a garden

Shakespeare often used the image of a garden to emphasise the need for top-down, linear control, including the need to 'prune', 'weed' and 'prevent the seeds of doubt' being sown.

But the garden is also often used as a metaphor for a living system that is alive with enabling, co-creative inter-activity. For example, in *The Garden of the Beloved* Robert Way used the garden metaphor to emphasise the symbiosis between flowers and bees, worms and earth. It shows the need for 'gardeners' to value different things and nurture saplings (as well as sometimes dealing roughly with 'weeds').

Implication of the image of a garden

Integrated care is like a garden in that it requires harmony between many different factors, and also control. The metaphor reminds us that control and harmony both have their place. Competition and collaboration both have their place in a beautiful 'garden'. It reminds us that shared leadership teams are needed to cross-pollinate ideas between different 'flowers'. It reminds us that thousands of everyday, unglamorous actions are needed in a healthy garden – watering plants, fertilising the soil, cutting paths, and so on.

Image – sailing at sea

Integrated care is like sailing at sea because you have to work with forces other than your own (unlike a car that has its own engine). To get where you want to go you rarely travel in a straight line – the best route comes from assessing the forces around you and using them to your advantage. You may need to change destination if your chosen one proves to be too difficult. You have to anticipate the resources you will need to travel in unfamiliar waters. You need to trust the resilience of your boat. Sometimes you go into port, to shelter from a storm.

Implications of the image of sailing at sea

The need to constantly adjust direction requires you to travel with optimism, paying attention to the winds of change, maximising opportunities and minimising the threats around you.

Image – music, dance and the performing arts

The performing arts are particularly revealing about people's ability to work as teams. A theatre group might have only a couple of rehearsals before they have to go on stage and creatively interact. Members of a choir or orchestra have to listen to each other's harmonies and adapt mid-breath to a change of beat. Dancers need to feel the sway in their partners' movements and subtly adapt to fit well together. Each of these requires listening, sensing and team-working, without necessarily using any words at all.

Taking part in music, dance and the performing arts teaches you to listen and appreciate different contributions to a team effort. In *The Power of Music*, Hallam summarises research into the effect of playing music on a child's developing mind. It causes a 17 per cent increase in retaining verbal information, increased confidence and increased social skills. One explanation for this is that it teaches a budding musician how to listen and adapt in response to others – to play well, musicians have to listen to themselves and to their fellow players, to the notes and to the tune. They must distinguish different melodies, harmonies and beats, and adjust their playing to enhance that of others.

She writes:

> there is compelling evidence for the benefits of music education on a wide range of skills including: listening skills which support the development of language skills, awareness of phonics and enhanced literacy; spatial reasoning which supports the development of some mathematical skills; and, where musical activities involve working in groups, a wide range of personal and social skills.

 Hallam, S. *The Power of Music*. Music Education Council, 2015. http://static1. 1.sqspcdn.com/static/f/735337/25902273/1422485417967/power+of+music.pdf? token=wEczWdwUkfdyHzLbWjuPZ06g2T8%3D

Implications of the image of music, dance and performing arts

Leaders of community-oriented integrated care need to listen to a wide diversity of opinion and subtly adapt their language to harmonise well with them. They need to recognise when people are saying similar things in different ways and help them to find a common language – a common tune. They need to help people to reframe what they are saying in ways that harmonise better with their shared endeavour. They need to recognise that merely taking part will, in time, increase skills of active listening and adapting to others.

Theories that help to engage with complexity

Theories are 'ideas intended to explain something, especially the general principles that can be applied in different contexts'. Medical science mainly uses a combative, linear theory of change, because of its need to fight diseases. This can inhibit the use of non-linear ideas of change that are more appropriate in dynamic and complex situations such as integrated care and health improvements. Here are four theories that help to make more subtle and complex actions in dynamic situations:

- Leadership as sense-making
- Health as positive narrative unity
- Evolution as complex co-adaptation
- Trusted relationships as a co-constructed sense of 'we'

Theory – leadership as sense-making

The image of the heroic leader – a charismatic figure that people blindly follow – has limited use in integrated care. It may be a useful posture when facing the cameras or in emergency situations, but in complex, changing situations, people need to think for themselves. Over-reliance on 'knights in shining armour' obstructs good practice. Instead, people need to make sense of things for themselves.

Weick argues that making sense of something makes it usable. Sense-making is concerned with things like: 'placement of items into frameworks, comprehending, re-dressing surprise, constructing meaning, interacting in pursuit of mutual understanding, and patterning' (p. 6). He argues that sense-making is more than interpretation. 'Sense-making is about authoring as well as interpretation, creation as well as discovery' (p. 8). He agrees with Thayer who analyses leadership: 'A leader at work is one who gives others a different sense of the meaning of that which they do . . . The leader is a sense-giver.'

 Wieck, K. *Sensemaking in Organisations*. Thousand Oaks, CA: Sage, 1995

Leaders are sense-makers when they help people to make sense of 'the woods and trees' in their personal and their work lives. Leaders, and leadership teams, remind people of the journeys they are making – their origins, destination and steps along the way. They help people to travel hopefully in a world that is full of surprises. They help people to transform their situations by reassembling the pieces to make better sense as a whole.

Sense-making is what peace-makers, team-builders and marriage guidance counsellors do. They help people to listen to each other, and appreciate their different perspectives. They help individuals and groups to make sense of things that were initially beyond their understanding. They help them to engage in shared adventures with a positive mindset, so that people change their ways of thinking. They start to see opportunities as well as threats. They discover ways to release the creative potential in their relationships.

Implications of the theory of leaders as sense-makers

The main job of leaders who are sense-makers is to help people to do things for themselves. It is not enough to be right; they must also find ways for other people to discover what's right for themselves. Leaders need to be skilled at sense-making and also helping individuals, organisations and systems to make sense of things.

Theory – health as positive narrative unity

Too often people use the term 'health' when they mean the absence of disease. Health is a positive thing – a sense of being alive in the moment. Healthy people are generous. They interact creatively with others. They rise above adversity. They adventure in optimistic ways.

Chapter 15 describes health as a 'positive narrative unity'. We are each the lead actors in the feature film of our lives, and support actors in the feature films of many others. To be healthy we must be fit enough to move our own stories forwards optimistically, rising above adversity and helping others to develop positive life stories.

This theory helps us to see beyond the problems of the immediate moment. It helps us to make sense of things in our lives that might seem to be contradictory.

Implication of the theory of heath as positive narrative unity

At any moment, it is difficult to see the sense of our emerging life stories. We have to trust the process and later, with hindsight, the story becomes clear.

Narrative unity allows us to locate dis-eases within a healthy life story. With this reframing, diseases can even *enhance* health when they stimulate someone to develop themselves in more meaningful ways – a near-death experience can be surprisingly empowering!

Narrative unity also reminds us that everyday modest actions can promote health. Merely showing interest in someone's life story is a health-promoting action – it makes people feel valued, listened to as a whole person beyond their diseases, and valued as part of a greater community. In narrative unity, simple things can be powerful – like remembering someone's name and the things they like. Smiles often work.

We can also promote health by helping people to make the connection between the person they wish to become and the actions required to get there. Everyday examples include reminding people of the link between smoking and potential future illness, of the damage done to relationships by insular and defensive attitudes, and of the importance of a good balance between work and play.

Narrative unity is valuable at all ages, but it is particularly obvious in elders. Reminiscence, advanced planning and music all help them to describe their life stories.

Theory – evolution as complex co-adaption

One conceptual difficulty is how past certainty and future uncertainty connect. The past is 'known' and the future is 'unknown' and to be created, so they are quite different kinds of thing. How research and development connect is pretty much the same question.

Two commonly held beliefs about how research (R) and development (D) connect are equally unhelpful in the context of integrated care and health promotion:

1   One belief expects research to directly lead to development; it believes that 'causes' lead to predictable 'effects', so 'evidence' should be applied blindly into practice.
2   The other belief is that the world is so complex and mysterious that research into the past has little relevance, so development can only happen by starting again.

The first belief puts 'R' above 'D' and the second puts 'D' above 'R'. Each might give people something to start with, but each, on its own, is misleading. The future and the past are connected, but not in linear ways.

If we think of the world as a *complex adaptive system* we see non-linear connections between past and future. Different people's past will contribute different things to what happens in the present and its interpretation. What emerges is usually a bit of many things. Like a baby – neither the father or the mother, but a creative fusion of both.

Nevertheless, many people in the Western world hold strongly to the belief that 'D' should follow 'R' in a direct, linear way. Scientific advances have created an illusion that everything can be controlled. Many are not aware that the relevance of research insights in other contexts cannot be assumed, nor that there are alternatives to the laboratory science.

The theory of a linear relationship between 'R' and 'D' has been attributed to thinkers from the 'Enlightenment' like René Descartes, Charles Darwin and Adam Smith. The writings of these giants of history suggest that they did not themselves believe in simple relationships between cause and effect. Descartes, to whom the theory of body–mind split has been attributed, believed in an all-powerful God who managed things to do with complexity, mystery and surprise. Darwin, to whom the theory of natural selection has been attributed, did not mean survival of the most ruthless, but of the most adaptable. Smith, to whom the theory of market forces has been attributed, lived in times when the market-place was a dynamic, creative, haggling place where collaboration and competition co-existed.

In one way or another, they all acknowledged that 'soft', organic co-adaptation is a natural aspect of the world, and at the same time 'hard', linear control is a natural aspect. The truth is a dynamic entwinement of both.

In recent years, the rise of *complexity theory* in science and *systems theory* in development has given rise to a new concept that is recognised by both – the *complex adaptive system.* The term has been particularly associated with Fritjof Capra, Ralph Stacey and Paul Plesk. It's an important term for integrated care because it provides a unifying language for researchers and developers. It also describes a mechanism whereby the past and the future become relevant to each other – through listening, learning and co-adaptation.

The 2010 Health Foundation Review of the ways in which the concept of Complex Adaptive System has been used in healthcare stated:

> Complex adaptive systems thinking is an approach that challenges simple cause and effect assumptions, and instead sees healthcare and other systems as a dynamic process. One where the interactions and relationships of different components simultaneously affect and are shaped by the system.

 The Health Foundation. Evidence Scan: Complex Adaptive Systems. August 2010. www.health.org.uk/sites/health/files/ComplexAdaptiveSystems.pdf

Implications of the theory of complex co-adaptation

The idea that everything is constantly changing in response to everything else explains why we need to set developments within a framework of collaborative learning and coordinated change – of participatory action research. This allows people to keep in touch with the changes in others, and co-evolve sensitively. Dialogue helps people to understand the rationale for change. Time and support help all to adapt to the emerging new reality. This is what learning organisations and learning communities do. They create 'R&D systems' in which research informs development (action) and development informs research, with ongoing participation of local people in the reflecting and acting processes.

Effective health-care systems use *connected learning spaces* to help people to stand back and reflect on evidence in the light of their experiences. They also pilot collaborative innovation to test out what it might be like 'for real'.

Theory – relationships as a co-constructed sense of 'we'

Integrated care is helped by trusted relationships. It begs the question: 'What is a trusted relationship?'

A mechanical answer is this: a trusted relationship is when someone takes their part reliably in their transactions with you – they will do what they have agreed to do. But health and community-oriented integrated care are concerned with more than transactional relationships. The organic, constructivist lens shows us that trusted relationships are *co-created* through interaction between people, so the people become in some ways entwined. This is a *spiritual* connectedness – something that happens at a deep inter-personal level and is neither the property of one nor the others. Sometimes it's called 'love'. It is a normal, everyday experience that is important because it binds people together in a profound way that can withstand difficulties and release co-creative energies. It produces motivation, innovation and resilience that functional relationships often lack. Its importance is often forgotten, perhaps because it can't easily be put into words.

Implications of the theory of relationships as a co-constructed sense of 'we'

High-performing teams need more than functional relationships. They need trusted relationships with a strength of bond and intuitive togetherness that produces motivation, innovation and resilience. Team players in community-oriented integrated care need to develop trusted relationships like this. We need frequent, repeated opportunities to develop such team players through shared projects that make people draw on their inner resources.

Methods that inform good decisions in complex situations

Kurt Lewin (1890–1947) was a German-American pioneer of social, organisational, and applied psychology in the United States (Chapter 19). He argued that neither nature (inborn tendencies) nor nurture (how life experiences shape individuals) alone can account for the behaviour and personalities of individuals. Instead, both nature and nurture shape each person.

He argued that the world we encounter is far more complex than we realise initially. It does not respond well to simple manipulation or to one approach to inquiry. This led to his famous quote: 'If you want to truly understand something, try to change it.' Lewin is particularly well known for his methods that help with visualising and working with the dynamic and complex nature of 'the real world'. His ground-breaking work on applied research led to the now everyday terms – 'action research', 'forcefield analysis', 'group dynamics' and an approach to change that he called 'unfreezing, change, freezing'.

Here are four methods that build from Lewin's thinking about how to see initially invisible patterns within complex situations:

- Rapid appraisal – brings together a range of information to see more of the whole
- Backwards mapping – imagines end goals and deduces the support needed to achieve them
- Systems mapping – a diagram of connections
- Action learning – cycles of learning and action

Rapid appraisal (see also Chapter 11)

To lead change in a complex situation you need to understand key aspects of the situation quickly, and then establish a network of people to transform it. *Rapid appraisal* is a good technique for doing this. It combines different kinds of insight to understand the story so far. It also engages those same people in action for collaborative improvements. It combines 1) literature, 2) observations and 3) interviews.

The first step is to decide on an open question that all the people you encounter are likely to have an answer to. It should be easy to answer and should aim to reveal insights into the desired change. Here are some examples:

'What system for diabetes care would be best for us?'
'How can we improve team-working in our practice?'
'What are the most important things to improve in our practice?'

Here are the next steps:

1 Read what other practices have done.
2 Observe what actually happens in your practice (e.g. behind reception and at a clinic).
3 Put your question to different people (including patients).

This approach will help you to understand what needs to change, the best thing(s) to do and who will most energetically support the changes. It helps to decide who should be in the shared leadership team to lead the changes.

As you learn more you can adjust your question or ask supplemental ones. You ask interviewees who else you should ask and what literature you should read, stimulating a 'snowball' of information.

Rapid appraisal helps you to draw a map of how things connect in the present system, and how they should connect in a future envisioned system (see systems mapping below). The leadership team can use the maps to discuss strategy. They ask informants to redraw the maps to better represent the present world and their future vision.

Rapid appraisal will help you to:

• Identify different roles in the present system and the forces that shape them
• Map relationships in the system and the meetings, projects, subgroups, alliances and networks that could be used to develop their relationships further
• Reveal a future vision that is broadly accepted by the stakeholders
• Anticipate future difficulties with achieving a shared vision

---

There are different models of rapid appraisal.

Rapid rural appraisal has been used by the World Health Organization to assess community health needs. In this model participatory researchers build an information pyramid that helps local people to see their whole context.

Rapid institutional appraisal has been used by the Open University Systems Department for staff induction. In this model, new staff members use semi-structured interviews and group work to understand the university, to identify developmental needs and to build relationships.

Rapid reconnaissance has been used in qualitative research to enter a research field quickly. In this model, members of interdisciplinary teams conduct informal interviews to produce an initial understanding of the whole situation.

Method – backwards mapping

A backwards mapping exercise reveals that environments, networks and facilitative leadership teams are often more effective than line management and protocols. It brings into view a full range of factors in the environment that enable success. For example, when a receptionist has to deal with an aggressive patient, it helps to pay attention to things that might prevent the aggression in the first instance, as well as how the receptionist responds. Similarly, a supportive team may be more helpful to the receptionist than the specific protocol she or he has to follow.

You start by focusing on a specific place in the system (e.g. patient–receptionist encounter). Then consider the environment that will encourage desirable behaviour. When you have done that, one layer back, consider the environment that will support that environment. If that's difficult to grasp, try this exercise.

Using a flip chart, write as clearly as you can what behaviour you think should happen at a *peripheral point*, for example in your practice's reception. Suppose you want receptionists to listen sensitively to patients who present and deal effectively with aggression. You also want them to answer patient's questions about appointments, prescriptions, local services and a range of long-term conditions.

Then imagine the range of things that will make this more likely to happen, one layer back, you examine ways in which the environment the receptionist works in can support the desired behaviour. This may lead you to consider:

1   Training and feedback about 'customer focus'
2   Immediate manager support for tricky moments
3   A hidden place to retreat to
4   Schedules of which clinicians are working, and when they are working
5   A handout or pack that helps patients to get the best out of your practice (e.g. prescription policy)
6   Updated list of local services on the waiting-room wall
7   Multidisciplinary teams to oversee different care pathways

Next, write down what the next layer should provide to support good outcomes. This may lead you to consider:

1   Leadership teams for various long-term conditions
2   A well-configured practice computer to present stream-lined information
3   Support for the patient participation group to update the waiting room wall
4   Action learning meetings to review issues

You continue looking at layers that support layers until you reach the most central place that you can influence.

Of course, receptionists are only one 'most peripheral point'. There are others – clinicians in consulting rooms, patients with acute illnesses, administrators of invoices, leaders of improvement projects. Backwards mapping can help to plan support for all of them.

The same approach can help to devise good steps in a long-term project, for example when making a project plan. You decide what you want to achieve and by when.

Then you ask what needs to be in place one step back in order to achieve your desired outcome. Then you work out what is needed one step before that, and so on. This process often reveals many things you should have done yesterday! But you can catch up.

Backwards mapping was described by Richard Elmore, a 1960s advisor to the American government. He observed that social change was much more likely to happen when the required behaviour at the most peripheral places was supported by layers of supporting structures, coupled with a central strategic coalition that represented, in a political place, the perspectives of the people at the most peripheral places.

 Elmore, R.F. (1979) Backward mapping: implementation research and policy decisions, *Political Science Quarterly*, 94: 601–616

Systems mapping

This involves drawing a map of how different things connect. There are different ways to approach the drawing. One is described in the Introduction to this book.

A systems map quickly shows how complicated most everyday situations are. It can quickly reveal why things don't work as well as they should.

A systems map does not have to focus on an abstract 'system'. It can focus on individual patients. Here is an extract from *Working Whole Systems* that explains how systems mapping was used in the context of large group interventions:

> Systems mapping enables participants to recognise the complexity of a system of which they are a part, and understand better how it works . . . We begin with an 'archetype' – a description of a situation whose essentials repeat themselves again and again, though not identically, as in a stereotype. For example a woman in her late 70s has a 'turn' at 10 pm one evening when she falls over and seems a little confused. . . . Participants describe how this situation might develop and this is mapped in public, on the wall. If participants have time and trust each other they will eventually begin to describe how things *really* happen rather than how they are supposed to happen.
>
> (p. 126)

 Pratt, J., Gordon, P. and Plamping, D. *Working Whole Systems*. London: King's Fund, 1999

When Head of the Open University Systems Department, Ray Ison used systems mapping to facilitate organisational change (personal observation). An illustrator would sit with one group and draw how that group imagined everything to connect. The illustrator would then take this drawing to another group and ask them to critique it, deriving a second systems map which would then be critiqued by all groups in iterative cycles until everyone agreed.

In workshops to explore ideas about complexity, Fritjof Capra used an illustrator to draw a map of the interaction of ideas between participants (personal observation).

Software can support systems mapping on a large scale. *Scenario Generator* is often used in the NHS to envision care pathways. It connects with real-life databases to imagine what will happen at each part of a care pathway, allowing cost and capacity to be calculated.

 Cordeaux, C., Hughes, A. and Elder, M. (2011) Simulating the impact of change: implementing best practice in stroke care, *London Journal of Primary Care*, 4: 33–37. www.radcliffehealth.com/ljpc/article/simulating-impact-change-implementing-best-practice-stroke-care

Action learning

Action learning involves inquiry (asking questions about the past), learning (reflecting evidence against experience) and action (doing something in the future). It requires *active listening* that picks up cues beyond the immediately obvious, to surface things that matter.

Models of action learning range from ad hoc encounters of clinicians in which they discuss a problem, to long-term action learning sets in which participants tackle current concerns.

Developing a live manual (Chapter 6), large group events (Chapter 10) and annual cycles of collaborative improvement (Chapter 5) all involve action learning. For example, you could set up a drop-in action learning set where participants share anecdotes about patient care and identify implications for practice. Or you could facilitate practice meetings to discuss the practical implications of audits, improvement projects and significant events.

In *ABC of Action Learning*, Revans explains why reflecting on perceived problems with work colleagues, and taking shared action for change, is essential in organisations like general practices which need to do more than 'express only the ideas of the past' (p. 3).

He argues that separating abstract knowledge from concrete action is unhelpful. Knowledge does not stand alone and needs to be applied. Revans writes: 'the distinction drawn by academics between research, action, learning and communication are highly artificial. There can be no action without learning and no learning without action' (p. 14).

 Revans, R. *ABC of Action Learning*. London: Lemos & Crane (Mike Pedlar Library), 1998

Exercise: use techniques that see parts and wholes

Use an organic image, theory or method that helps to see the connection between parts and wholes in your case study. Does it help you to see what is going on? Does it help you to see what to do?

Chapter 8

How to run meetings that make sense of multiple perspectives

Key message: Community-oriented integrated care needs meetings at which people from different backgrounds learn from and with each other.

In this chapter:

- Stakeholder workshops help people to learn and change
- Good facilitation is needed
- Leadership styles at meetings – chairing, facilitating and story-holding
- Rehearse
- Think in threes
- Small-group–large-group oscillations
- Compose yourself
- Techniques that stimulate creative interaction between participants:

  o Beginning a meeting – getting people ready to take part
  o Envisioning – help participants to build shared vision
  o Illuminating steps in the journey
  o Surfacing hidden connections
  o Rehearse real-life situations
  o Team roles
  o Continue discussions in other places

- Transformational change takes time
- Exercise: assess your developmental needs

Stakeholder workshops help people to learn and change

> All the world's a stage. And all the men and women merely players. They have their exits and their entrances. And one man in his time plays many parts.
>
> (Shakespeare, *As You Like It*)

Sooner or later you will need to bring many people together to share insights and negotiate ways forward – probably sooner.

Simply getting a practice manual for diabetes agreed will need at least one meeting where the various people needed for success contribute their ideas. You will miss important insights if you forget to do this. At such meetings people listen to each other, develop shared vision and build relationships. This begins to develop them as a team or community that can be further built upon at future meetings. Well-run meetings give a sense of theatre in which participants co-create the way forwards, creating a sense of ownership and shared purpose.

They are not meetings of the committee type. They are more like workshops that generate new insights from multiple-way conversations. They are particularly effective when embedded into annual calendars. This helps people to take part in them strategically. You can use them strategically too, for example to develop shared leadership teams and to support cycles of inter-organisational improvement.

This chapter describes how to design these meetings. Some well-established models of *large group events* are described in Chapter 10.

Good facilitation is needed

Chapters 5 and 9 describe annual cycles of inter-organisational improvement that enable large numbers of people from different disciplines to engage in collaborative activity. The annual cycle includes a series of connected events at which participants learn from and with each other, co-design projects and as a result come to trust and understand each other better. This chapter describes how to design and lead those meetings for maximum effect.

Successful meetings enable participants to revisit their past stories and potential shared future. Participants leave affirmed of their own value, with renewed understanding of their shared journey, with new insights and new friendships.

Facilitators use techniques that allow many different points of view to be treated seriously and to be woven into a broader narrative. The techniques help to understand why the different participants think and behave the way they do.

Facilitation helps people to see the ways in which their insights and actions could complement each other. It is what marriage guidance counsellors and diplomats do. They get people to stand back from their own concerns to see things from other points of view; then try small collaborative experiments to explore how to be mutually enhancing.

But beware – facilitators are rarely thanked and often blamed. When it works, people believe they did it themselves; and when it doesn't they need a scapegoat. You have to have a sense of humour. You need your own network of support.

PAUSE: What skills would you like to learn about leading meetings?

Leadership styles at meetings – chairing, facilitating and story-holding

To lead successful meetings you need to move with ease between three different styles – chairing, facilitating and holding the story. Most meetings benefit from a bit of all three, adjusted according to the expectation of participants, the time available and the purpose of the meeting. If you prefer one particular style, it is worth practising the others.

Chairing

Discussions move *to and from the chair* in direct, linear ways. This approach is useful to explore facts and perspectives one at a time. You can use it to keep an agenda moving along quickly, to avoid potentially harmful interaction between participants, and when the topic of discussion might not benefit from creative discussion.

Facilitating

Discussions move *between participants* in a fluid flow of ideas, prompted by the *facilitator* (rather than 'chair'). This approach is useful for building relationships, creating new ideas and shaping consensus. This style is enabling, helping people to communicate and do things for themselves. As a sole method it can seem slow, but for co-creative issues it often gets people to where they need to be faster than more controlling approaches.

Story-Holding

At the beginning of a meeting the chair reminds the group of the story so far, and at the end summarises its progress. In between, she/he marks new developments in the story. In this style the leader helps participants to see their shared journey.

Rehearse

Backwards mapping (Chapter 7) helps you to plan the agenda. You start with what you want to have achieved by the end of the meeting, then work backwards, to plan each stage. This approach helps to work out how much time to allocate to each stage. Mentally rehearsing each stage of the meeting with your team will help the meeting to unfold in your mind's eye and also help everyone to make sure that it stays 'on track'.

The more complicated the meeting, and the more you aim to achieve, the more it is important to rehearse. Check the sound system. Sit in all the chairs to check there are no obstructing pillars or distracting noises. Feel what it is like to be in those chairs as a participant. Are the chairs too close? Or too far apart? Do you want them in rows or café style? Walk through the meeting to rehearse movement from one stage to another. Make sure that you have enough catch-up time in the later part of the meeting.

Before the meeting, draft a timeline of activities anticipated afterwards. This may change as a result of the meeting itself, but thinking about it in advance will make you more aware of the kind of thing you expect to happen, and the elbow room you have to manoeuvre.

At every meeting remind participants of the meetings they need to attend in the future – as far ahead as you can.

Think in threes

Three is a good number if you want people to think beyond their personal concerns to see broader issues. Thinking about one or two issues encourages reductionist, polarised or oppositional thinking; thinking about four or more issues can overwhelm them.

You can ask three questions in a buzz group, programme three cycles of feedback in a workshop, organise three linked workshops, resource three annual cycles. You can build momentum by linking the trio of activities thoughtfully, so each one builds on the others, or enhances them in some way. The facilitator can help people to see their relevance of all three by linking them to their shared story. Linking to the story is especially important if the story is easy to forget (for example when the events are far apart).

When planning a sequence of three questions or exercises in the same meeting, start broad and then focus. Start and end with positive ideas, sandwiching the negative. Move from participants' personal experiences, to more abstract ideas, then to practical plans.

For example, when directing a 20-minute buzz group on priorities for the year, with tables of four to eight people, you could say:

On your tables please answer the three questions that are written on your sheet:

1   List the things that are going well that you want to keep.
2   List the things that are not going well that you would like to change.
3   List your top three proposals for this year's improvement project.

In 20 minutes we will ask you to feed back into the room one answer to the third question, each table in turn. Please choose an answer that is different from previous tables. We will keep going around the room again until all ideas have been aired.

Small-group–large-group oscillations

When designing a workshop programme, oscillate between focused and broad issues, relating both to the evolving story by starting with the past and moving towards the future.

A simple format with broad application is moving between small-group discussion in side rooms (4–12 participants) and large-group plenaries. A sequence of questions is asked and answered in the small groups and fed back at plenary session.

A similar approach uses 'buzz groups' of two to eight without leaving the plenary room.

For example, the following programme is likely to hold together a whole workshop in a health network when considering a proposed innovation in a local health community:

a)   Aims of the day including the overall question the participants want to answer and the story so far, e.g. developing care plans for patients with complex conditions
b)   Round of introductions, each participant explaining their key insight into the question (on separate tables if there are too many people to do it as one group)
c)   Small group session one – what are the implications for clinical consultations?
d)   Plenary feedback distilling key agreements and disagreements
e)   Small group session two – what are the implications for general practices?
f)   Plenary feedback distilling key agreements and disagreements
g)   Small group session three – what are the implications for the whole system?

h) Plenary feedback distilling key agreements and disagreements
i) Plenary discussion to agree next steps and people to lead them

Compose yourself

During a meeting, remember that people cannot see how nervous you feel if you choose not to show it. You will look more confident if you cut out apologies and do your best not to feel defensive. Better to look humble and calm, than anxious or arrogant.

By all means rehearse your lines as much as you like before the event, but work from bullet points at the event itself. You can use notes or a visual aid to make it look effortless. Interact with the audience with your eyes, smiles, gestures and quips. They help people to feel that you are all on the same side.

You aim for participants to leave at the end understanding more and feeling motivated to take part in the next stage.

It does not matter if the plan changes – a sense of ownership by participants is often more important than following the original plan exactly. In any case, the world has a curious way of working out well, despite deviating from the planned path. Often you win more in the long term when you lose in the moment.

Getting the right level is important. Too simple and people become bored; too advanced and people lose the thread. Getting the right level requires good preparation. Inviting participants to put forward examples from their experiences helps to find the best level.

Get used to gauging the energy in the room, speeding up or slowing down depending on the 'buzz'. After a few meetings consider a new meeting format.

It is important to show that you are not merely listening, but *actively listening*. You can demonstrate this by appropriate interjections – checking out what someone has said by repeating it back to them, nodding at key places, responding quickly and appropriately to something that somebody says.

Generally speaking, humour and appreciative asides catch people's attention in a good way. But you have to know your audience, and appreciate the limits of your own skill!

Active listening, team-working, struggling to understand others, skilled negotiation, being on top of the story – these are things that impress people, in a good way.

Techniques that stimulate creative interaction between participants

You can find techniques in books and websites that can help to keep people creatively engaged in a meeting. You can also make your own up or get the group to generate them. Best to see beyond the technique to see what it is trying to achieve:

Beginning a meeting – getting people ready to take part

*   Agenda, story, aims., e.g. remind everyone of the story so far
*   Energisers, e.g. one thing that puts a smile on your face; throwing a ball to others to continue a stream of ideas

- Ground rules, e.g. 'I statements', 'mutual respect', 'listen', 'keep time'
- A round. e.g. participants in turn say something useful for the agenda

Envisioning – help participants to build shared vision

- Visioning and guided imagery, e.g. talking people into a semi-meditative state, or drawing a visionary future on the wall
- Life-mapping, systems mapping, mind-mapping, conversation-mapping, e.g. Tony Buzan's Mind Maps
- Wants and offers – participants describe their roles, what they can offer other participants and what they want from others

Illuminating steps in the journey

- Feedback progress of projects, e.g. teams give the audience an update of progress
- Cross-pollinate ideas between different leadership teams, e.g. invite participants to pick out from each other's presentations things they could learn from
- Digital stories – a three-minute update in electronic form, including images, music, videos and words

Surfacing hidden connections

- Nominal grouping and hexagons – participants write a different idea on each hexagon or sticky square and post them on a wall to build categories
- Brainstorm and rainbowing – throwing out ideas without comment and later clustering them into rainbows of ideas
- Force-field analysis and complex power diagram – things that help and hinder progress and things that influence other things

Rehearse real-life situations

- Role play, scenarios and simulations – individuals and groups play different roles to set up a creative dynamic
- Goldfish bowl – people observe without comment as other people interact within a circle of chairs
- Real-time strategic change – a scenario that is 'real' in that people are playing their own genuine roles

Team roles

- Theatre, music, art, e.g. write a play that describes the local story
- Team-building exercises, e.g. outward-bound exercises
- Preferred styles, e.g. 'the kind of animal I am', Belbin roles in groups, Honey and Mumford learning styles, Myers Briggs personality types

Continue discussions in other places

- Interactive bulletins – a bulletin asks a question and invites replies; it publishes them in the next bulletin and asks a new question, and so on
- Web-based or e-mail discussion, e.g. 'chat rooms' and moderated discussions
- Cascading conferences – conclusions from one conference are cascaded to the next

Transformational change takes time

Facilitators need to remember that learning and change rarely happen immediately. They happen between events, rather than at them. Meetings may simply start people thinking and give them options to find out more. But deeper learning happens off stage, when people later reflect quietly on what they have experienced – another reason why we need ongoing cycles or inter-organisational learning and change.

Individuals need to change their ways of thinking about relationships from being controlling and hierarchical, to being equal and co-creative. Some find this very hard. Even in one small organisation you must not expect too much too soon, so chart a long-term course.

You may find it helpful to think of your work as planting seeds to be grown by others on another day.

Exercise: assess your developmental needs

Go through the Appendix – a curriculum for leadership of community-oriented integrated care. List the skills you want to develop within one year and within five years. List the skills you want your teams to develop.

Part III

Integrating care and promoting health from geographic localities

In Part III:

Who might find Part III useful?

Part III is written primarily for those who lead and evaluate integrated care and health promotion in geographic areas. Leadership might come from a coalition of general practices, public health, community services, faith groups or local authorities. A geographic area is a good place to lead integrated care and health promotion because when people work in the same area they can often agree on the main health issues. Also it is easier to collaborate when participants do not have to travel far. On the other hand, it can be difficult to get people to engage because they are often preoccupied with their own concerns.

Success needs a properly resourced facility to bring people together. Stakeholders need to feel confident that engaging will be a good use of their time. This means that participants should find the meetings valuable, engagement give benefits to their organisations and the collective action causes measurable improvements in the health of local people.

Applied research units and leadership courses (Chapter 4) can help leadership teams to:

a) Engage stakeholders in annual cycles of learning and change
b) Facilitate stakeholder events
c) Evaluate overall effects
d) Have effective ways to retain personal balance in the midst of it all

The image to support Part III: Case studies of local health communities

On the left hand are geographic localities (50,000 population works quite well in UK cities). They are called *health networks* when they collaborate for medical purposes (e.g. care pathways or education), and *local health communities* when they collaborate more broadly for health improvements. This includes developing the skills of local people to interact positively with others. Each can be a case study of community-oriented integrated care.

Inside each locality, multidisciplinary leadership teams facilitate annual cycles of participatory action research that help local people to collaborate for health improvements. Team members come from different parts of health services – generalists, specialists, public health; and from other sectors – schools, faith groups, social services and voluntary groups.

Any number of research and improvement projects can take place at the same time, within and between localities. Routinely gathered quantitative data (e.g. hospital admissions and surveys) and qualitative data (e.g. patient stories) are aligned to localities. These can evaluate the collective impact of multiple interventions on well-being, citizenship, capacity and economics. At stakeholder events, local people discuss the data in the light of their experiences to agree a story of what is happening.

In the middle of the image is a sequence of large group events at which representatives of case studies and strategic partners meet to review data from case study sites and from other places (e.g. stakeholder surveys). This helps them to learn how to improve the sites and also generate broader insights into policy. Each event builds on previous

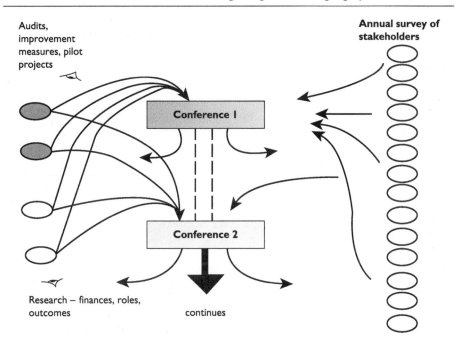

Figure III Case studies of local health communities

ones, helping to describe collaborating sites as *comparative case studies* that unfold over time. The overall effect is a 'R&D System' – research informs development and development informs research in never-ending cycles of inquiry, learning and change. It builds trust between participants from which comes a sense of community. It builds a network of activists beyond locality boundaries that facilitates cultural change towards collaborative working.

Strategic connection of such *learning spaces* can stimulate learning and change throughout large areas – whole cities, whole systems and more.

Introduction to Part III: integrated care needs team-working and systems-thinking

Community-oriented integrated care is complicated. Acute illness is the simplest – you treat it or trigger the care pathway. Care for minor long-term illness is also fairly straightforward – similar things happen every week.

Shared care for long-term conditions and for multiple illnesses is more complicated. It requires care plans, self-help and care teams whose members dip in and out when needed.

Health promotion is the most complex. It aims to achieve:

- Healthy citizens skilled at self-help and healthy lifestyles
- Socially and environmentally aware citizens able to build and sustain relationships
- Resilient communities able to 'think globally and act locally'
- Cost-effective public services

Achieving all of this does not mean that local people simply apply the models of others. It means creating a powerhouse of learning, collaboration and innovation throughout local communities. Thoughtful local discussion understands and appreciates diverse perspectives. It brings into view bigger pictures and whole systems of care. This bottom-up knowledge-generating activity must link with top-down policy to provide both 'vertical' and 'horizontal' dialogue, challenge and sharing of intelligence. It creates a learning system, a 'R&D System'. This is not a linear idea. It is an idea that life naturally evolves through co-adaptation, often with unexpected outcomes. We must abandon the idea that isolated projects, direct force or individual leaders have the power to cause integration. Instead everyone needs to become skilled at synchronicity, mutuality, connectivity. This is how to facilitate cultural change, trusted relationships and positive co-evolution.

In other words, what sustains integrated care and integrated health promotion is creative interactions between groups and individuals as they shape and lead projects. Individuals need to be skilled at this, as team players who respect different perspectives. Organisations need to apply principles of *organisational learning*. *Learning networks* need to link *learning communities* where openness to learning and change is the cultural norm. *Boundary-spanning leadership teams* need to engage people from all parts of the relevant systems in the co-design of system-wide improvement projects.

Different sections of this book show how to do this:

- Part I describes policy for whole system team-working.
- Part II describes how to lead a series of collaborative projects from local organisations such as a general practice.
- Part IV describes how a combination of machine and living system images helps to see dynamic interactions as well as concrete structures.
- Part V describes how to stimulate shared adventures that build team players.

This part (III) describes how to lead integration from perhaps the most powerful place of all – geographic areas where people feel they belong. *Local communities for health*.

Southall Initiative for Integrated Care

Between 2009 and 2012 the *Southall Initiative for Integrated Care* in west London piloted a *local health community* with 23 general practices in a geographic area of 65,000 population, subdivided into four localities each with about six general practices.

Cycles of collaborative reflection and coordinated improvement led to the co-design of five improvement projects. Different localities piloted different projects. These addressed problems of integration between primary care and other services – mental health, acute care, social care and community care. For each project a multidisciplinary leadership team was formed that included practitioners from general practices and relevant specialties.

The projects were:

1   Implementing the Ealing dementia strategy, including early diagnosis and ongoing monitoring of patients (not published)
2   Developing community links for the support of children and families (not published)
3   Implementing the diabetes strategy, including diabetic clinics in general practice

Unadkat, N., Evans, L., Nasir, L., Thomas, P. and Chandok, R. (2013) Taking diabetes services out of hospital into the community. *London Journal of Primary Care*, 5: 2, 87–91, DOI:10.1080/17571472.2013.11493386

4   Treating anxiety and depression in black and minority ethnic populations

Evans, L., Green, S., Sharma, K., Marinho, F. and Thomas, P. (2014) Improving access to primary mental health services: are link workers the answer? *London Journal of Primary Care*, 6: 2, 23–28, DOI:10.1080/1757 1472.2014.11493409

Evans, L., Green, S., Howe, C., Sharma, K., Marinho, F., Bell, D. and Thomas, P. (2014) Improving patient and project outcomes using inter-organisational innovation, collaboration and co-design, *London Journal of Primary Care*, 6: 2, 29–34, DOI:10.1080/17571472.2014.11493410

5   Aligning data from various computer systems to locality boundaries

Stoddart, G., Gale, R., Peat, C. and McInnes, S. (2011) Using routinely gathered data to evaluate locally led service improvements, *London Journal of Primary Care*, 4:1, 38–43, DOI:10.1080/17571472.2011.1149332

They gave rise to other papers in which the authors reflected on lessons arising:

Chandok, R., Unadkat, N., Nasir, L., Evans, L. and Thomas, P. (2013) How Ealing health networks can contribute to efficient and quality healthcare, *London Journal of Primary Care*, 5: 2, 84–86, DOI:10.1080/17571472.20 13.11493385

Dhillon, A. and Godfrey, A. R. (2013) Using routinely gathered data to empower locally led health improvements, *London Journal of Primary Care*, 5: 2, 92–95, DOI:10.1080/17571472.2013.11493387

Chapter 9

Engaging people in cycles of inter-organisational learning and change

Key message: To develop a local community for health, leadership teams in geographic areas need to engage large numbers of people in ongoing collaborative activities.

In this chapter:

- Geographic localities allow shared developmental space
- Developing a local health community requires repeated 'freeze–unfreeze'
- How to motivate people to engage in collaborative activities

    o   Make it easy – through facilitative infrastructure
    o   Make it effective – with methods that help to engage with complexity
    o   Make it make sense – with a science of co-evolution
    o   Make it fun – with skills to travel hopefully

- Make the rationale for participation clear
- Make the leadership clear
- Make the steps clear
- Develop networks of leadership teams through linked leadership courses
- Exercise: engage stakeholders

Geographic localities allow shared developmental space

Geographic areas provide *shared development space*. Large numbers of organisations can align their activities to the same area and, by linking them, have collective impact greater than the sum of their individual contributions. This also builds community spirit. This is why leading integrated care and health promotion from geographic areas can be so effective.

One difficulty is getting people to sustain a collaborative approach. Everyone is preoccupied with their own concerns. People often do not understand or even like each other. There may be past hurts to reconcile. People project their anxieties onto others, fuelling conflict and subverting progress. Many ignore the need to refresh relationships, and they drift apart.

Local collaboration for care and health improvements is not always realistic.

This chapter explains that you can sustain relationships in a community by helping people to dip in and out of each other's lives to co-design small but useful things.

Annual cycles of collaborative learning and coordinated action help to do this. They remind people that they are connected to others and need to co-evolve. Locality leadership teams lead these cycles, support the projects that emerge and incrementally develop the localities as *local health communities*. An applied research unit can train the teams and facilitate networks of such teams to stimulate integration throughout much larger areas.

A local health community differs from a health network by focusing on collaboration for whole population health, and not merely the treatment of diseases. They are localities that are small enough to feel you belong and large enough to have political impact. In London and Liverpool (UK) we have found that a good size has been 30–70,000 population (3–20 general practices; 17–40 full-time GPs). This size allows people to feel a sense of intimacy that contrasts with a sense of anonymity that often prevails in larger areas.

Leading change in a locality is rewarding because transformational change can happen in a reasonable period of time – years rather than decades or generations. You can experience how your personal input makes a difference. You can value the goodwill and intelligence that participants bring to the table, and sensitively deal with the obstructions that they can introduce. You can get an instinctive feel of what is achievable at different stages.

Developing a local health community requires repeated 'freeze–unfreeze'

Developing a community is not easy. People are often unfamiliar with collaborative processes; they can be slow to engage and quick to leave. You will quickly recognise that direct control is of little value, but may lack experience of other approaches. You may feel overwhelmed by the number of conflicting factors. Change will be constant. There will always be something obstructing progress. Unexpected crises will throw you off balance. And the more you succeed, the more people will believe that they did it themselves. In the process, you might become confused about who you are and what value you are adding.

Leaders of integrated care and integrated health promotion within geographic localities need to engage many different individuals and organisations in coordinated activities. You can do this through a sequence of events, planned long in advance, that review the shared vision, co-design steps towards that vision and take small but useful collaborative steps towards it.

This process is called 'freeze–unfreeze'. You get people to stand back and imagine where they are heading (unfreeze) and design the route. Then they focus on getting tasks done (freeze) before they again stand back to review progress and design next steps (unfreeze).

There is some merit in just getting going and seeing what happens – fresh-faced enthusiasm is a motivating factor of its own. So you should not be frightened of just getting on with it. But you will need to plan if you are to succeed in the long term.

Long-term success needs careful planning because much can go wrong. Even spectacular success can cause your downfall. Your participatory approach may conflict with a more controlling approach of others, causing misunderstanding and even conflict. There may be too few people to share leadership roles, and you may burn out. You may become too skilled and inhibit others. The infrastructure you set up to sustain progress may be incompatible with that of the broader system. Short-term success can easily lead to long-term failure.

So, make plans at the outset for both short-term and long-term success, and renew the plans frequently. As well as planning the processes of engagement, plan to retain political support and nurture your personal networks of support.

The clearer you are about the resources you will need in a few steps time, the more able you will be to seize opportunities to get them. Clarity about resources will also help you to avoid carelessly abandoning vital infrastructure by failing to recognise its importance.

How to motivate people to engage in collaborative activities

For people to reach out of their 'silos' to collaborate for the sake of the system as a whole they have to get something out of it for themselves. Idealism is not enough (though it helps). Payment is not enough (though it helps). Liking people is not enough (though it helps). For example, improvements in quality, pursuing a personal interest, being part of a 'happening' team and developing useful skills can all motivate people to engage.

When the commitment is clear and realistic it is easier to persuade people. So we need to make engaging easy, effective and fun. We have to make sure it makes sense too.

Make it easy – through facilitative infrastructure

Part I (*policy for integrated working*). Four chapters describe **infrastructure** that makes it easier for people from different backgrounds to collaborate for care and health promotion:

- Developing localities as healthy communities makes horizontal integration easier
- Three-tier system of shared care makes vertical integration easier
- Seasons of activity make it easier to align the activities of different disciplines
- Applied research units can solve problems, broker partnerships and support networks of leadership teams to make all aspects of collaboration easier

Make it effective – with methods that help to engage with complexity

Part II (*integrating care from small enterprises like general practice*). Four chapters describe **methods** that make collaborative activity effective:

- Annual cycles of inter-organisational improvement help useful projects to emerge
- Live manuals help individuals to contribute effectively to whole system initiatives
- Dynamic images, theories and methods help to make sense of complex interactivity
- Group learning techniques help to run effective meetings

Make it make sense – with a science of co-evolution

Part IV *(understanding community-oriented integrated care and health promotion)*. Four chapters describe a **science** of dynamic interactivity and holistic co-evolution:

- Community-oriented integrated care is important and feasible
- General practitioners are sense-makers who cover all aspects of health and disease
- Health is being alive in the moment and not merely the absence of disease
- Evaluation of complex interactivity needs to reveal hidden connections and emerging shape, as well as established facts

Make it fun – with skills to travel hopefully

Part V *(community-oriented integrated care and health promotion – making it work)*. Four chapters describe the **skills** we need to journey with others in optimistic and enjoyable ways:

- Social network theory shows how to coordinate collaborative adventures
- Transactional analysis shows how to develop happy relationships
- Learning organisations build strong teams
- Strategic partnerships help all citizens to contribute to health and care

Make the rationale for participation clear

Community-oriented integrated care needs long-term mechanisms that help people from different parts of the system to get to know each other and undertake small collaborative projects. You may find it difficult to persuade people that these relationship-building mechanisms are needed, especially when they think of integrated care only as a machine.

A key argument is the need to continually build trusted relationships across organisational boundaries. Integrated care is more than a machine. It is also a network of relationships.

People work well together when they have trusted relationships. It is not so easy to get people to collaborate when they lack them. Indeed it is common for individuals and teams to find fault with those they do not understand, and even manufacture conflict. As is often said: 'the trouble with teams is they are always looking for other teams to play against'. This is how 'silos' develop – people who have something in common develop a shared identity and micro-culture, becoming internally supportive and externally combative. They form clubs, gangs, teams, disciplines and communities with self-defined boundaries. The boundaries will inhibit integration and reinforce fragmented care if there are no mechanisms to cross them.

The ease with which people form 'silos' that fragment care explains why integrated care needs mechanisms to repeatedly stimulate relationships across boundaries – vertically in care pathways and horizontally within and between communities. You need to maintain these mechanisms and audit their use.

When people co-design improvements rather than merely agree with someone else's design, the sense of ownership motivates them to sustain and further improve the changes. Over time, this transforms the way they think – to see themselves as active participants within a living system, rather than mindless cogs in a machine. A useful methodology to achieve this sense of ownership is participatory action research (PAR) (Chapter 11). PAR stimulates cycles of learning and change that will, over time, develop and sustain a culture of participation and collaboration. Maintaining the infrastructure to support these cycles is important to enable new people to engage, and to develop innovation in organic ways.

The following chapters help to explain the rationale for a participatory approach:

- Chapter 13 explains why community-oriented integrated care needs participation
- Chapter 19 explains that participation is a learning organisation principles
- Chapter 11 explains that PAR can include different approaches to evaluation

Make the leadership clear

- Chapter 3 explains that leadership teams can facilitate PAR within 'seasons of activity' to align activities of multiple organisations.
- Chapter 4 describes different kinds of leadership team that should inter-connect:
  o *Practice leadership teams* oversee developments within a general practice
  o *Locality leadership teams* lead developments within a locality
  o *Project leadership teams* lead projects
  o *System leadership teams* lead developments throughout a whole system
  o *Oversight teams* critique and shape the plans

Make the steps clear

Chapter 3 describes seasons that help to synchronise shared care, health promotion and PAR initiatives. The same seasons help to integrate care from a health network or local health community. For example:

November–December: season of reflection

A *system leadership team*, supported by an *oversight team* facilitates a November/December stakeholder workshop at which participants:

- Decide the improvement initiative(s) for the coming year
- Identify research question(s) for the initiatives
- Agree a project or *system leadership team(s) to lead the project(s)*
- Agree *practice leadership teams* and an *oversight team*

January–March: season of planning

The *project or system leadership team*:

- Meets regularly
- Forms a database of stakeholders
- Draws a connections diagram

- Undertakes a rapid appraisal for each project
- Holds a training workshop (February)
- Provides monthly updates for the *practice leadership teams*

April–July: season of coordinated actions

The *project/system leadership team*:

- Supports updating of care plans for the coming year
- Facilitates two stakeholder workshops (April/May and July)
- Provides monthly updates for various other teams and key contacts

August–October: season of concrete experience

The *system leadership team*, *practice leadership teams* and *oversight team* make the planned changes.

November–December: season of reflection

System leadership teams and oversight team:

- Facilitate a November/December stakeholder workshop
- Re-draw the diagram of how the people would connect in the new system
- Start the whole sequence again

Develop networks of leadership teams through linked leadership courses

Individual team members encourage the participation of individuals and organisations who know and trust them. Together the team has broad reach. A network of leadership teams has even broader reach, potentially a powerful force for change throughout whole systems.

Leadership courses can develop shared leadership teams from different places, learning from and with each other. Each course can strategically involve teams from different parts of a system to facilitate integration throughout that system. This is what Lambert did in the 1990 team-building workshop programme (Chapter 10). Such a course needs to:

a) Provide a learning space within which participants from different teams cross-pollinate ideas and update each other on progress
b) Introduce participants to the theory and practice of integrated care and leadership of whole system learning and change
c) Support the development of comparative case studies and writing for publication
d) Use principles of real-time strategic change (Chapter 10) to link local developments with strategic development of much larger areas (e.g. local authority boroughs, clinical commissioning group boundaries, or whole cities)

Networks of such courses could cross-pollinate ideas across much larger areas, with things like exchange programmes and shared projects – whole countries, whole continents.

Exercise: engage stakeholders

Write a strategy to engage different constituents in the annual cycle of learning and change in your case study.

Chapter 10

Large group events help people to creatively interact

Key message: Stakeholder events help to build local health communities.

In this chapter:

- Whole-system events help people to co-evolve creatively
- Whole-system events are like street carnivals
- Origin of whole-system events
- Future Search conference
- Appreciative inquiry
- Open Space Technology
- Real-time strategic change
- Team-building workshop programme
- Exercise: hold a whole-system event

Whole-system events help people to co-evolve creatively

You will need to bring large numbers of people together again and again in order to re-agree their shared vision, review progress and develop new initiatives. Without opportunities to re-engage with each other, people will drift apart.

This chapter describes some well-established models of *large group events*. They help people of different backgrounds to meet, exchange opinions and learn about each other, develop shared vision and coordinated action plans and build relationships. This helps them to develop themselves as a learning network or learning community.

Whole-system events are like street carnivals

Whole-system events are exciting, dynamic events. Like street carnivals they provide interconnected ways for participants to be creative with others.

Like a carnival, a whole-system event provides what Handy described as an 'Empty Raincoat' – a space you can use for your own purposes; for multiple purposes.

 Handy, C. *The Empty Raincoat*. Reading: Arrow, 2002

Like a carnival, a whole-system event engages a wide range of people in creative interactions at the level of their interest. It permits self-organisation. Different 'music' in different 'rooms' attracts and deters different people, so organisers provide signposts, maps and timetables that help people to navigate the whole event. Ground rules help people to creatively engage – ground rules like 'listen', 'smile' and 'reach out to others'.

Like carnivals, preparation is time-consuming – programmes, refreshments, performers, facilitators all need to be coordinated. The better the planning, the more it seems as if no planning was done. Another similarity with carnivals – participants leave at the end with smiles on their faces and a lot of mess to clear up!

Origin of whole-system events

In 1997, Bunker and Alban described large group interventions that helped businesses in the US to foster vision, energy and commitment in their employees.

They identified 12 models. These large group interventions enabled hundreds or thousands of employees to interact in coordinated ways to express themselves within a bigger system (the company), and from this re-form their sense of collective identity. They also explained the origins of large group theories in the twentieth century – gestalt psychology (e.g. Kurt Lewin), systems theory (e.g. Von Bertalanffy) and psychoanalytic psychology (e.g. Wilfred Bion).

 Bunker, B and Alban, B. *Large Group Interventions*. Jossey-Bass. San Francisco, CA: Jossey-Bass, 1997

In 1999, Pratt, Gordon and Plamping used five of these models in UK cities to facilitate whole system change – *system mapping, Future Search conference, appreciative inquiry, Open Space Technology* and *real-time strategic change*.

 Pratt, J., Gordon, P. and Plamping, D. *Working Whole Systems*. London: The King's Fund, 1999

They explain that events are best designed with the metaphor of a *living system* in mind. The metaphor helps the designers to see the dynamic activity needed to integrate different approaches and build webs of relationships that bind people together within it.

They wrote:

> [Living systems can] repair themselves . . . continuously order themselves and retain an identity . . . Ordered but not controlled.
>
> (pp. 13–14)

> Sufficient numbers of the people involved must recognise that their futures are linked, that they are part of an ongoing interdependent system.
>
> (p. 126)

> Whole system events may be designed especially to meet the needs of a particular situation. Or the design may start from one of the well-tried designs for large group intervention that is then modified appropriately.
>
> (pp. 125–6)

They also explain that designing the event in a collaborative way is often the most effective thing – more than the event itself. If you want to devise your own event, go to Chapter 8.

Event Title	Useful to	Participants	Duration
Future Search Conference	Explore past, present and future to conclude shared vision and collaborative plans	60–70	2½ days
Appreciative Inquiry Meetings	Guide a multidisciplinary team or advisory group when moving forward a set of issues over time	4–12	10–12 x 2–4 hours
Open Space Technology	Explore a set of problems for which there may be multiple complementary 'answers'	25–200	1–3 days
Real-Time Strategic Change	Repeated encounters between different groups with different managerial and clinical leadership roles	Any number	½ day repeated over time
Team-building Workshops	Develop a network of leadership teams	Five teams of 5–12	2½ days

The table lists a few models that might be useful in health care. A brief description of each follows to give you a sense of what they practically entail. You don't have to follow the exact script of these models. You can devise your own format. Chapter 8 describes a range of techniques that you can use.

Whole-system events can be embedded into annual calendars. They can be led by sequential cohorts of shared leadership teams that move things on in between events.

Future Search conference

Future Search helps a diverse group of people to explore their past, present and desired long-term future, and conclude short-term coordimated actions towards their shared vision.

 Weisbord, M. and Janoff, S. *Future Search: an action guide to finding common ground in organizations and communities*. San Francisco: Berrett-Koehler: 2000.

Future Search could be used to develop a community around a cluster of general practices and health centres. It could be used to develop a coordinated plan to address a social concern such as violence, a medical concern such as diabetes or other 'wicked problems'.

It is optimal to have 60–70 participants. The 'sponsor' creates a cross-stakeholder planning group and together they agree the conference focus and dates. They identify and approach potential participants.

Wiesbord and Janoff describe eight conditions for success:

1   'Whole system' in the room
2   Whole 'elephant' as context for local action
3   Common ground and future focus, not problems and conflicts
4   Self-managed small groups
5   Full attendance
6   Healthy meeting conditions
7   Three-day event ('sleep twice')
8   Public responsibility for follow-up

The 'sleep twice' condition is based on the learning principle that reflection is essential for learning. It is not the number of hours studying that causes success, but the number and depth of learning cycles, that include quiet time to reflect on what you have learned.

In the three days, participants:

1   Review the past
2   Explore the present
3   Create ideal future scenarios
4   Identify common ground
5   Make action plans

In the first afternoon participants map their memories on a wall of paper. Long strips of 'butcher' paper line the walls with titles 'Personal', 'Global', and X (conference focus) (p. 18) each with date-marks every 5–10 years. In small groups, participants discuss memories, global trends and other patterns. Participants in each group are a cross-section of the whole conference. They first record these on group flip charts and then write them on the butcher paper, and explain them to the whole conference using a microphone. This is how the collective memories are captured for all to see. This work takes about 2½ hours.

The second task uses Buzan's concept of a 'mind map' to explore the external trends that are having an impact on the conference topic (p. 88). Participants are asked to 'come on down' to the paper. A *diagrammer* writes the name of the conference topic inside a circle (e.g. Santa Cruz County). Using a microphone different people in turn describe a trend, such as 'increased environmental awareness'. The diagrammer writes this as a thread emerging from the central circle, with a concrete example written beside it. The group debates each new trend to decide if it is a branch from a previous idea or something new. As more and more ideas are put forward, the collective mind map becomes a complex display of interconnected issues. Participants physically touch the map to feel part of it.

 Buzan, T. and Buzan, B. *The Mind Map Book*. London: BBC, 1995

Before people break at the end of the first day they post seven sticky dots on the trends they consider most important for the conference. Different disciplines or stakeholder groups have different coloured dots to indicate which groups care most about which trends. Unfinished tasks or issues are acknowledged before finishing for the day.

At the start of day two participants have a close look at the wall and have an open discussion about it. Then they break into uni-disciplinary groups to draw personalised versions of the mind map. This clarifies the different concerns of different stakeholders.

In these stakeholder groups they also take part in a 'prouds and sorrys' exercise, in which they identify things they are proud of, and sorry about.

Before lunch on the second day the mixed groups of the first day reconvene to explore their shared hopes for the future. They are invited, as 'scenario groups', to put themselves 5, 10 or 20 years into the future, 'imagining that they have made their dreams come true'. They are asked to list on flip charts a) concrete examples of what 'had' actually happened, and b) the major barriers they had to overcome on the way (p. 99).

In the afternoon the scenario groups present their shared visions of the future to the whole conference in any way they like – drama, skit, play, TV and so on. Each scenario group then writes on three flip charts:

1   Common future – 'what we all agree about' (e.g. value statements and abstractions)
2   Potential projects – 'how to get what we want' (e.g. concrete proposals, policies)
3   Not agreed – recognising conflicts that have not yet been worked through

When the lists are finished, scenario groups pair up and then merge their two sets of flip-chart work into one. All lists are posted on the wall. Each idea on the combined lists is cut into a 'strip' – one idea on each strip. This gives a mass of agreed ideas that can contribute to the next stage of developing a consensus.

On the morning of the third day, participants group the strips into themes and discuss whether this is a true reflection of their consensus. The rest of the day is taken up with two rounds of action planning from the consensus, starting with the stakeholder groups. The sponsor has the last word.

Cross-organisational planning groups move things forward until the next event.

Appreciative inquiry

Appreciative inquiry often works from a problem that is important to a range of stakeholders – for example, road traffic accidents or elderly care. To examine the chosen situation, it brings together diverse groups of people to work out how to build from the *best* in an organisation or community. Approaches range from mass-mobilised interviews to a large, diverse gathering called an appreciative inquiry summit.

Whatever the specific methods used, it uses a '4-D' cycle:

• Discover individual and collective motivation and meaning (e.g. sharing stories)
• Dream a vision for a transformed future (building from the best of what is)
• Design a plan based on the envisioned future (e.g. in small groups)
• Manifest a destiny based on learning from ongoing action (including evaluation)

Whitney and Trosten-Bloom explain that:

> The 4-D Cycle of AI is based on the notion that human systems, individuals, teams, organisations and communities grow and change in the direction of what they study.
>
> (p. 6)

> As a process of positive change, AI is fully affirmative.
>
> (pp. 10–11)

> The role of an Advisory Group is to lead the organisation into a calculated leap into the unknown.
>
> (p. 109)

They describe eight different 'Forms of Engagement' (p. 31), of which one, 'Progressive AI Meetings' (p. 45), may be useful to guide the actions of shared leadership teams that keep things working between larger stakeholder events.

 Whitney, D. and Trosten-Bloom, A. *The Power of Appreciative Inquiry.* San Francisco: Berrett-Koehler, 2003

Open Space Technology

Open Space enables self-organising groups to deal with complex overlapping issues and develop sets of coordinated action plans.

 Owen, H. *Open Space Technology: a user's guide.* San Francisco: Berrett-Koehler, 1997

Open Space Technology can be used by a local health community to help organisations explore their potential contributions to a shared effort for care or health promotion. For example, it might explore improving care of the elderly or reducing drug abuse.

This method allows hundreds of people to self-organise. It is especially good at exploring problems that everyone agrees are important, but for which no one has 'the answer', or for which there may be multiple complementary 'answers'. It helps different disciplines or organisations to develop simultaneous and complementary projects.

It can take one to three days. 'In one day the conversations will be stimulating and intense. In two days, that conversation will be recorded for posterity. With three days, priorities can be established and next steps identified' (p. 26).

Participants first stand in a circle in a 'market place of ideas'. Whoever wishes steps into the middle and describes a discussion group they would like to convene. Anyone who wants to join the discussion group can then do so. 'Groups of 25–50 have about 30 issues, groups of 100–200 have about 75 issues' (p. 104). They write their name and the issue on a piece of paper on the 'wall' – the 'community bulletin board'.

Participants 'buzz' around the 'wall' that includes the daily schedule. The pieces of paper are posted on a 'space/time matrix'. A few sessions are combined and some change times to avoid clashes, but for the most part the schedule is fixed fairly quickly.

Then everyone goes to the groups of their choice – about 90 minutes per group session.

The group convenor writes up notes of the meeting on a computer there and then, with headings like 'Title', 'Convenor', 'List of Participants', 'Discussion & Recommendations'. These summaries are posted on the 'wall' and become part of the conference report.

It requires microphones for the plenary sessions, one break-out room per 20 participants, one flip chart per break-out in geographic areas room, marker pens, sticky squares and masking tape, and one computer per 20 participants. Refreshments are available continuously.

Owen attributes the success of these events to 'creating time and space, and holding time and space' (p. 57). The facilitator is 'totally present and absolutely invisible'.

The 'rule of two feet' allows people to go wherever they like when they like. 'Bumblebees' constantly flit between one group and another, often cross-pollinating ideas. 'Butterflies' do very little as 'centers of non-action' (p. 100), but somehow cause significant conversations – 'perhaps significance emerges precisely because no-one is looking for it'.

Owen advocates four signs posted in prominent places (pp. 72–73):

1   Open Space Theme (briefly stated)
2   The Four Principles:

   • Whoever comes are the right people
   • Whatever happens is the only thing that could have
   • Whenever it starts is the right time
   • When it's over, it's over

3   The One Law: The Law of Two Feet
4   An Exhortation: 'Be prepared to be surprised'

The community assembles twice a day – for morning announcements and evening news. This simple structure provides a flexible space for self-organising.

Real-time strategic change

Real-time strategic change is often used to transform large organisations and could be adapted to transform whole systems of care. It can be used to facilitate repeated encounters between different health-care groups with managerial and clinical roles.

As with all whole-system event models, designing it takes a long time. The design process is often more important than the event itself.

Any combination of large group event formats and techniques (Chapters 8 and above) can be used. For example, it can involve debate between existing leadership groups as though in a role play or goldfish bowl. The distinguishing feature is that the people who are role-playing are the same people who actually hold those roles. In other words, they are 'role-playing' their real roles. This can help people to deeply appreciate the constraints of others. It also stimulates everyone to feel that they are on the same side.

After one stage of debate the various groups go away to rethink their positions. They lobby other groups and negotiate offstage. Then they reconvene in a series of encounters (potentially over years) to transform their shared story incrementally.

For example, commissioners and providers could engage in such a process. So could health and social care leaders, or physical and mental health practitioners. In 'role' they are allowed to take issue with each other forcefully, yet they remain appreciative and supportive in reality. A listening and constructive approach is enhanced by the moderating effect of facilitators and other participants.

Team-building workshop programme

This model was created in the 1980s by Deryck Lambert, then at the UK Health Education Authority. It was designed to develop multidisciplinary team-working in general practices, especially in the development of health promotion clinics (e.g. heart health, diabetes).

Five general practice teams of 5–12 individuals of different disciplines go on a residential workshop for two and a half days (i.e. three nights' sleep). They are facilitated to undertake a series of activities out of which emerges their detailed practice plans and also a great deal of understanding about team-working. Before and after the workshop, the facilitators visit the practices to support the team to develop the practice.

The effect on the teams and the local health system is enhanced by a 'local organising team' (LOT). The LOT organises the workshops. It includes members of key support organisations that provides a 'horizontal', 'boundary-spanning' network of practitioners and managers that help to align the agendas of their organisations and stimulate next steps in local policy.

This model may be valuable for GP federations to develop a network of practice leadership teams, or for local health communities to develop as case studies of integrated care.

Exercise: hold a whole-system event

Hold a whole-system event led by a shared leadership team.

Chapter 11

Structured inquiry – an important ingredient

Key message: Research, audits and service improvement projects influence local policy when they are embedded within annual cycles of locality improvement.

In this chapter:

- Research, audit and evaluation should use a full range of inquiry methods
- Inquiries provide snapshots of evolving stories
- Fourth-generation evaluation
- Participatory action research
- Reframing audit and evaluation as fourth-generation evaluation has many benefits
- Research methods categorised by paradigm of inquiry
- Case studies
- Rapid appraisal
- Using routinely gathered data to evaluate case studies of integrated care
- Exercise: pilot research methods

Research, audit and evaluation should use a full range of inquiry methods

Collaborative working in geographic areas needs research, audit and evaluation to assess progress and inform policy. The table shows how the NHS Health Research Authority (HRA) distinguishes these different kinds of inquiry to decide whether a project needs research ethics committee (REC) governance (that oversees research). The HRA defines research as a study that derives 'generalisable new knowledge'. This means knowledge that is intended to be applied in other contexts.

Audits and service evaluations generate knowledge for local learning. They need to be governed by local institutions. Audits check if things are happening as planned. Evaluations assess the merit of a new way of doing things. The HRA has no authority over them. It includes them in its guidance simply to avoid people wasting the REC's time with projects intended for local quality improvement.

The column on research includes qualitative as well as quantitative research. Traditional ('quantitative') approaches to inquiry (positivism) need to be complemented by 'qualitative' approaches that see relationships (critical theory) and processes of relationship-building (constructivism). Insights from each of these traditions are valuable. In complex, dynamic situations all are needed because they reveal different aspects of the whole.

The columns on audit and service evaluation, however, use solely the language of objective, quantitative science – 'measures', 'standards and 'judgements'. This is not enough for community-oriented integrated care and health promotion. As with research, we need qualitative insights when auditing and evaluating complex and emerging phenomena – for example we need to know if an innovation has had unexpected consequences.

Leaders of audit and evaluation should be prepared to use a full range of inquiry methods. In complex situations they should routinely use a combination, and set them within processes of local learning and change. This is what Guba and Lincoln argue. They call it 'fourth-generation evaluation'. This chapter presents Guba and Lincoln's argument, then categorises established inquiry methods into the three paradigms of inquiry described in Chapter 16.

A table for researchers and reviewers to use (modified from published literature)

Research	Clinical audit	Service evaluation
The attempt to derive generalisable new knowledge including studies that aim to generate hypotheses as well as studies that aim to test them.	Designed and conducted to produce information to inform delivery of best care.	Designed and conducted solely to define or judge current care.
Quantitative research – designed to test a hypothesis. Qualitative research – identifies/ explores themes following established methodology.	Designed to answer the question: 'Does this service reach a predetermined standard?'	Designed to answer the question: 'What standard does this service achieve?'
Addresses clearly defined questions, aims and objectives.	Measures against a standard.	Measures current service without reference to a standard.
Quantitative research – may involve evaluating or comparing interventions, particularly new ones. Qualitative research – usually involves studying how interventions and relationships are experienced.	Involves an intervention in use *only*. (The choice of treatment is that of the clinician and patient according to guidance, professional standards and/or patient preference.)	Involves an intervention in use *only*. (The choice of treatment is that of the clinician and patient according to guidance, professional standards and/or patient preference.)
Usually involves collecting data that are additional to those for routine care but may include data collected routinely. May involve treatments, samples or investigations additional to routine care.	Usually involves analysis of existing data but may include administration of simple interview or questionnaire.	Usually involves analysis of existing data but may include administration of simple interview or questionnaire.

(continued)

(continued)

Research	Clinical audit	Service evaluation
Quantitative research – study design may involve allocating patients to intervention groups.	No allocation to intervention groups: the health-care professional and patient have chosen intervention	No allocation to intervention groups: the health-care professional and patient have chosen intervention

Source: NHS Health Research Authority: http://www.hra.nhs.uk/news/dictionary/ (accessed 10 May 2016)

Inquiries provide snapshots of evolving stories

Chapter 16 explains that inquiries from the positivism and critical theory schools imagine that facts are really there ('realism') and do not change. Of course they *do* change over time. Inquirers know this, so they repeat research at later dates to see what has changed. What they are seeing are not eternal truths, but snapshots of stories-in-evolution.

However, the power of scientific inquiry to build machines can lead people into the mistaken belief that the world is a simple machine, whose components do not change and can be studied without considering other connected factors. This misunderstanding gets in the way of understanding anything dynamic, including integrated care and health promotion. It gets in the way of doing good research, good audit and good evaluation in primary care.

So inquiry is less digging out unchanging facts and more illuminating real-life situations in a way that identifies a) superficial facts, b) hidden connected factors and c) evolving stories. A person may be unhappy (fact), be grieving and in debt (hidden connected factors) and incrementally transforming his/her life story to be more positive and coherent.

We need an approach to inquiry that brings these different approaches together.

Fourth-generation evaluation

Few have done as much as Egon Guba to analyse paradigms of inquiry. He orchestrated the authoritative analysis of the epistemology, ontology and methodology of positivism, critical theory and constructivism described in Chapter 16.

 Guba, E,G (ed.) *The Paradigm Dialog*. Newbury Park, CA: Sage, 1990

Few have done as much as Yvonna Lincoln in documenting what qualitative research is in its own right, rather than defining it as anything that isn't quantitative. With Norman Denzin she edited the 1994 and 2000 editions of the *Handbook of Qualitative Research*. They revealed a growing recognition that qualitative inquiry should not merely be an exploratory phase of a more important quantitative phase. Instead different qualitative traditions *think differently*, and reveal *different kinds of aspect* of reality. Reality is more complex, adapting and interconnected than any research approach can ever reveal on its own.

 Denzin, N.K. and Lincoln, Y.S. (eds) *Handbook of Qualitative Research*. Thousand Oaks, CA: Sage, 1994

 Denzin, N,K. and Lincoln, Y.S. (eds) *Handbook of Qualitative Research*, second edition. Thousand Oaks, CA: Sage, 2000

Guba and Lincoln, who were also life partners, teamed up to write *Fourth Generation Evaluation*, an elegant analysis of the history of evaluation in the US and UK. It shows how ideas about evaluation mirrored the development of positivist, critical theory and constructivist schools of thought. They first describe three generations from the positivist and critical theory schools:

1   **Generation of measurement:** From 1897, the positivist idea that truth comes in self-contained packages irrespective of context led to measuring things of stand-alone value – for example scores for intelligence and suitability for jobs.
2   **Generation of description:** Soon after the First World War the critical theory idea that different truths are inter-dependent led to a new evaluation approach. This approach first described the aims of an organisation (e.g. a children's school) and then assessed whether it did indeed achieve its aims.
3   **Generation of judgement:** From 1973, combined positivist and critical theory thinking was to be found in evaluation approaches that graded organisations (e.g. schools) in order of merit, using a range of scores.

 Guba, E.G. and Lincoln, Y.S. *Fourth Generation Evaluation*. Newbury Park, CA: Sage, 1989

They argue that all three generations are too objective and mechanistic. The authors state: 'all three generations overly rely on the methods of traditional science . . . and this results in "context stripping"' (p. 36).

They then describe how a fourth generation – 'responsive constructivist evaluation' – could reveal 'myriad human, political, social, cultural and contextual elements'. It involves setting inquiries inside a broader process of stakeholder review that helps local people to make better sense of their own stories – and help them to learn and change.

Guba and Lincoln conclude novel features of fourth-generation evaluation (pp. 253–256):

•   A socio-political process
•   A joint collaborative process
•   A teaching/learning process
•   A continuous, recursive and highly divergent process
•   A process with unpredictable outcomes
•   A process that creates reality

They state: 'The term *"findings"* has to be discarded since it suggests the existence of objective "truths" . . . The reconstructions that emerge from an evaluation are the literal creation of the participants and stakeholders who create them.'

To integrate the first three generations of evaluation with the fourth, their roles need to be redefined (pp. 259–262):

•   The first-generation *technician* is converted into a *human data analyst*
•   The second-generation *describer* becomes an *illuminator and historian*
•   The third-generation *judge* is a more humble *recommender of improvements*

Community-oriented integrated care and health promotion needs all four generations – the first three set inside the fourth. The fourth includes cycles of learning and change that allow participants to consider data from the first three and also their lived experiences. Through discussion they make sense of it all as a whole, to inform next steps.

Participatory action research (PAR) is a methodology that can combine all four generations of evaluation.

Participatory action research

Here is Foote Whyte's definition of PAR:

> Some of the people in the organisation or community under study participate actively with the professional researcher throughout the research process from the initial design to the final presentation of results and discussion of their action implications.

 Foote Whyte, W. *Participatory Action Research*. Newbury Park, CA: Sage, 1991

And here is an extract from a paper that describes our use of PAR in health care:

> PAR introduces the idea of a research community in which people of different backgrounds puzzle together about a research question. Participation of people who have different perspectives is particularly valuable when complex and contested phenomena are involved.
>
> At the start of a research project, participants with different insights can challenge the original assumptions of the researchers and produce a better research question than was conceived initially. At the stage of data gathering, different participants can help access different places. At the stage of acting on findings, the ownership gained through participation encourages complementary kinds of implementation.
>
> Ongoing conversations between different perspectives can also generate new knowledge and stimulate innovation by helping participants to see their own context with new eyes and test out new things based on these new understandings.
>
> Commonly, PAR does not answer one single research question but involves a series of inquiries about a real-life development that concerns a research community. Research questions are framed after the community has reflected on the findings of a previous cycle, producing 'spirals of self- reflective cycles of planning a change . . . observing the consequences of the change . . . reflecting on the consequences . . . re-planning'.

 Thomas, P., MCDonnell, J., McCulloch, J., While, A., Bosanquet, N. and Ferlie, E. Increasing capacity for innovation in bureaucratic primary care organisations: a whole system participatory action research project. *The Annals of Family Medicine*, 2005, 3: 312–317

Fourth-generation evaluation and participatory action research are methodologies that allow a community of inquirers to make sense of a range of evidence in the light of their lived experience, and translate these into practical action. This approach is increasingly used in health care using the term 'experienced-based co-design' – people with different backgrounds come together to reflect on data in the light of their personal experiences, and from this co-design and co-evaluate whole systems of care.

 Experience-based co-design toolkit. King's Fund. December 2013. https:/www. kingsfund.org.uk/projects/ebcd (accessed 31 December 2016)

Reframing audit and evaluation as fourth-generation evaluation has many benefits

Reframing audit and evaluation as fourth-generation means setting them within a framework of participatory action research. This accommodates the fact that every-thing in the world is continually adapting to everything else, despite having some features that seem to stay the same (they change slowly). Co-evolution is both unavoi-dable and desirable. Different perspectives on this constantly changing process help to get a rounded view.

Fourth-generation makes the changing nature of the world overt. It reframes inquiries as snapshots of broader stories-in-evolution. Here are implications for audit and evaluation:

- **Audit:** Instead of merely monitoring progress of the past, an 'audit' would consider new things that are developing. A multidisciplinary group would review the story of a service so far, including its expected trajectory, and perhaps invite others (e.g. in a focus group) to suggest a set of measures to illuminate the next stage of the story. Later, the results would be considered by a similar focus group, to establish if things are progressing as intended, and also to consider emerging directions.
- **Evaluation:** Advocates of a proposed intervention would be required to explain the rationale for its importance in the context of the evolving local story. Instead of evaluating an innovation in isolation, evaluation should consider the broader system(s), perhaps with a *rapid appraisal* or *large group event*. An *oversight team*, that includes different perspectives, reviews sets of innovations in the light of the organisation's story, and considers implications as a whole, including unexpected consequences.

A full range of research methods should be used in audit and evaluation, to be faithful to their purposes as described by the NHS Research Authority – 'to produce information that informs, defines and judges the delivery of best care'. They should study things like team-working, organisational coherence and patient empowerment as well as mechanical aspects. Such inquiries should be reviewed by a range of stakeholders to validate conclusions.

Reframing audit and evaluation as fourth-generation inquiry is helped by an applied research unit. This supports a local system of governance that ensures that good questions are asked, inquirers are trained, inquiry methods are rigorously following, and findings are used to stimulate local collaborative reflection and coordinated action.

Reframing audit and evaluation in this way has considerable advantages:

1 Locally led inquiries will be more rigorous, use more insightful inquiry methods, and have better impact on local policy.
2 Leadership of audit and improvement projects will be a training ground for research and development that individuals and organisations could lead at a later stage.
3 Locally led inquiries and research projects can be intertwined, developing research communities with university partners for student placements and research recruitment.
4 It will help to develop local health communities as case studies that measure the effect of innovation on broad issues, including wellbeing, citizenship, capacity and economics.

Research methods categorised by paradigm of inquiry

Different paradigms of inquiry (Chapter 16) make different assumptions about the nature of the world. Each shines a different kind of light to reveal different aspects of the whole, in the same way that a red light picks out red things and a blue light picks out blue things:

• Positivism assumes that truth comes in discrete packages that can be plotted on a bar graph. It sees individual things in isolation.
• Critical theory assumes that truth clusters into systems and networks of truth which can be represented on a mind map. It sees relationships between different things.
• Constructivism assumes that truth is a moment of becoming that can be woven into an emerging story. It sees the development of relationships.

In this section, research methods are categorised by the paradigm to which they most obviously relate. Rich insights come from a combination – for research, audit and evaluation.

Positivism

This produces individual measures that can be plotted on a *bar graph*.

Experiment

Compares data from two different ways of doing something. An audit could involve a patient recording the itch they experience on each leg when using different creams. An evaluated service improvement could count the number of patients who saw the same clinician after adopting a system for continuity of care. A research project could measure hospital readmissions of patients before and after patients have care plans.

Survey

Asks a series of questions (e.g. by post, email or website); for example do patients have a copy of their hospital discharge summary, what they think of the diabetic clinic, or if they want electronic access to their records. Surveys can ask open, qualitative questions as well as focused, quantitative ones.

Critical theory

This produces interconnected insights that can be linked on a *mind map*.

Focus group

A facilitator/moderator asks a selected group their views about something and allows them to refine their views through discussion; for example how a practice should work with carers to support self-help. A family conference to plan end of life care is a form of focus group.

Observations

Watching something and taking notes, looking for a range of specific things; for example patients passing through reception and the type of questions asked.

In-depth interview

Asking a series of qualitative questions, often using a semi-structured interview with prompts, for example people's views on the future of integrated care.

Correlations

Correlation research uses different kinds of data (e.g. surveys, experiments and observations) to consider if seemingly separate variables are related in some way - for example between retirement and death, or social networks and diabetes control.

Delphi technique and nominal grouping

A Delphi researcher sends participants a sequence of surveys, asking them to score statements that are then amalgamated and fed back to participants in repeated rounds. Nominal Grouping involves participants generating their own ideas then placing them under broad headings decided by the researcher.

Constructivism

This produces shared stories that participants know to be true because they contributed to the development of the stories.

Role play/scenarios

A group of people take different roles in a 'similar-to-real-life' situation. For example, one group role-plays funders of projects; it interviews (role-playing) funding applicants. It can include goldfish bowls and design groups that allow participants to see how others think when having to make sense of the information they are receiving.

Real-time strategic change

Similar to role play but people are 'playing' their own jobs (Chapter 10).

Constructivist grounded theory

Different ideas (e.g. on sticky squares) are moved around to form clusters of ideas. The process of interpretation is carried out by a group rather than researchers (as in traditional grounded theory). The interpreting can be done in a large group event such as Future Search or Open Space (Chapter 10). You simply invite participants to write their ideas on separate sticky squares and then move them around to collectively co-create new ideas.

Literature review

Systematic review (positivism)

The researcher searches the published literature using key terms relevant to their inquiry.

Snowball (critical theory)

The researcher asks informants what literature they think is important to consider in respect of the inquiry. The researcher then follows up the references used in those papers, continuing this until no new references are found.

Narrative (constructionist)

This involves discussion between people who are knowledgeable about different bodies of knowledge. Each explains why different papers and concepts are important to gain complementary insights into the question being asked. The different sets of papers are then obtained and key references that they quote are also pursued.

All three paradigms combined

1   Participatory action research (above)
2   Case study
3   Rapid appraisal

Case studies

The NHS Health Research Authority explains that a case study:

> focuses on a single unit of study; this may take the form of a single patient, family, ward or organisation. The researcher may use a mixture of methods to collect information about each case. Case studies can be used as examples of good practice or even to demonstrate when things have not gone so well.

 NHS Health Research Authority. http://www.hra.nhs.uk/news/dictionary/ (10 May 2016)

Robert Stake agrees. He explains that a case study can mean different things:

> Case study is not a methodological choice but a choice of what is to be studied . . . We could study it analytically or holistically, entirely by repeated measures or hermeneutically, organically or culturally, and by mixed methods – but we concentrate, at least for the time being, on the case.
>
> (p. 435)

> A case study is usually organized around a small number of research questions . . . information questions . . . themes . . . Issues are complex, situated, problematic relationships. They invite attention to ordinary experience but also to the language and understanding of the common disciplines of knowledge . . . A contract is draw between researcher and phenomenon [in order to ask] what can be learned here, that a researcher needs to know.
>
> (p. 440)

> Some call for letting the case tell its own story. We cannot be sure that that a case, telling its own story will tell all or tell well . . . The choices of presentation styles . . . are realistic, impressionistic, confessional, critical, formal, literary and jointly told.
>
> (p. 441)

 Stake, R.E. Case Studies. Chapter 16 in Denzin, N.K., Lincoln and Y.S., (eds) *Handbook of Qualitative Research*, second edition. Thousand Oaks, CA: Sage, 2000

An argument developed in this book is that local health communities should be case studies of community-oriented integrated care, including health promotion. Data can be aligned to these areas to evaluate the overall effect of multiple initiatives and collaborative working. By gathering data in the same way different sites can become *comparative case studies*.

When using comparative case studies it is important that mutual learning is the prime goal. As Stake cautions, leaders of comparative case studies can easily forget this:

> Researchers report their cases, knowing they will be compared to others . . . I see comparison as actually competing with learning about and from a particular

case . . . a research design featuring comparison substitutes the *comparison* for the *case* as the focus of the study.

(p. 444)

One critique of Stake's stance is that the same is true of all research methods. Every context is different so individual facts can mean different things. Different models will fit more or less well depending on local factors contexts. On the other hand, researchers *can* conclude interesting aspects to discuss, and from this conclude general principles of success.

Robert Yin emphasises this point, explaining that: 'Case studies are generalizable to theoretical propositions and not to populations or universes' (p. 10).

 Yin, R.K. *Case Study Research*. Thousand Oaks, CA: Sage, 1994

As long as we remember this warning that comparisons will mislead if the context is misunderstood, comparative case studies can be useful. We must use them to stimulate cross-site learning, rather than decide which is better or worse. Participants need to become skilled at telling their stories in rich detail, in the way that travel documentaries often do. Leaders need to be skilled at listening more than telling, understanding more than blaming.

Case studies can be revisited again and again to build a story that reveals generalisable principles of success. For example, the Peckham Experiment was a UK case study that was revisited between 1926 and 1950. It arose from rising public concern over the health of working-class people and increasing interest in preventative social medicine. The Pioneer Centre in South London paid 950 families a weekly sum (5 pence) to take part. The families had access to a range of activities such as physical exercise, swimming, games and workshops. Members underwent a medical examination once a year, and evaluation demonstrated sustained improvements in health. This led to the general principle that public health and primary care need to work closely together.

Participatory action research and case studies are not the only ways to build a rich picture of an area. For example, *community diagnosis* provides 'building blocks' of information; and *rapid appraisal* gains multiple perspectives by asking the same question of different people.

Rapid appraisal (also described in Chapter 7)

This is a good way to quickly get a range of insights into a complex situation.

It is used in developing-world countries to help local communities to see the complexities of their own situation, in preparation for coordinated action for change.

It is a form of *action research* that brings together information from different perspectives. The leader(s) of a rapid appraisal first define a simple but broad question that helps people to see connections within a whole system, and how the connections contribute to quality.

They then use interviews, observations and literature from a broad range of sources to answer the question. Rapid appraisal can be used in ambitious projects for whole-town or system-wide transformation. It can also be used in a contained, modest way, such as staff induction, or even as a way to simply strike up interesting conversations.

You first pose a question, for example:

- **Communication:** How do different members of the health-care team communicate, and how can this be improved (e.g. day and night, specialist and generalist practitioners, doctors and nurses)?
- **Infrastructure:** What things help people from different parts of a system to provide the best integrated service? And what things hinder?
- **Care pathways:** What do different disciplines contribute to end-of-life care? Safeguarding? Care plans? And what helps them to do this well?
- **Training:** What kind of training helps practitioners from different parts of a care pathway to do their job well? And how could this be improved?
- **The future:** What is the future service needs of patients? What are the workforce implications?

To answer the question, you:

- **Read literature** (a formal literature search or something less ambitious)
- **Interview a range of people** with insight into the role (e.g. a range of different disciplines who are information-rich). You can use a snowball approach to find them (ask each person you come across who else you need to interview)
- **Observe situations,** taking notes of things that illuminate your question. As far as possible describe objective facts rather than subjective judgements
- **Write it up** – as a report for local discussion or as a published paper.

Using routinely gathered data to evaluate case studies of integrated care

Comparative case studies of community-oriented integrated care and health promotion need data that can be compared between sites year-on-year. They need a facility for people in the sites to make sense of data in the light of their different experiences and contexts. They need a facility for people from different sites to consider the transferable lessons.

Data can be aligned to organisations such as general practices (adjusted for things like patient numbers), local health communities (adjusted for things like poverty), boroughs (adjusted for things like infrastructure) and countries (adjusted for things like wealth).

Data needs to give insight into the impact of interventions in the case study on *well-being, citizenship, capacity* and *economics*. Here are some measures to consider:

Related to demographics (perhaps impact on capacity and well-being):

- Age, poverty, morbidities
- Ethnicities and languages
- Standardised mortality ratios
- Use of public and private services
- Employment

Related to disease outcomes (perhaps impact on well-being and economics):

- Disease control (e.g. diabetes – Hb A1C)
- Complications of disease (e.g. amputations)
- Profiles of diseases and death rates
- Suicide and self-harm

Related to primary/specialist integration (perhaps impact on citizenship and economics):

- Unplanned admissions to hospital
- Place of death
- Shared care records accessed and updated by different practitioners
- Clinical problems solved through e-mail and telephone advice lines

Related to care plans (perhaps impact on well-being and citizenship):

- Care plans completed and updated
- Care plans used by others (e.g. out-of-hours practitioners)
- Discussions of care plans and changes as a result
- Patient/Family involvement in care plans

Related to collaboration (perhaps impact on capacity and citizenship):

- Locality meetings and their outcomes
- Changes in community and hospital referrals
- Locality innovation
- Self-care and health promotion courses

Related to whole-system quality (perhaps impact on capacity and economics):

- Patient and staff satisfaction
- Recruitment of staff
- Cost of care
- Additional resources secured

PAUSE: What things would you like to evaluate in your case study?

Exercise: pilot research methods

Use a range of research methods to illuminate aspects of your case study.

Chapter 12

Maintain inner peace

Key message: To avoid losing sight of who you are within complex activity, leaders of community-oriented integrated care need strategies to maintain their inner peace.

In this chapter:

- Leading integrated care can disturb your inner peace
- Three different ways of losing inner peace
- Things that help to maintain inner peace:

  o Maintain inner peace by retaining *narrative unity*
  o Maintain inner peace by retaining *confidence in your vision*
  o Maintain inner peace by retaining *control*

- Self-actualisation
- Travel hopefully
- Exercise: devise a personal plan for self-actualisation.

> If—
>
> If you can keep your head when all about you
> Are losing theirs and blaming it on you,
> If you can trust yourself when all men doubt you,
> But make allowance for their doubting too;
> If you can wait and not be tired by waiting,
> Or being lied about, don't deal in lies,
> Or being hated, don't give way to hating,
> And yet don't look too good, nor talk too wise
> (Rudyard Kipling)

Leading integrated care can disturb your inner peace

Leading integrated care means listening deeply to others and valuing their perspectives. This can cause you to lose sight of who you are. Strands in your plan can develop lives of their own that subvert your overall plan, making you feel trapped by your own vision. You may feel like a reed bending in the wind and fear that you will break; or have actually broken. The sheer number of things to do and people to relate to can make you feel overwhelmed. It is easy to lose balance on the merry-go-round of life. It is easy to lose inner peace.

Trusting the processes of co-adaptation and accepting *good enough* rather than perfection will help you to keep balance. If you have set things up in good faith, planned to the best of your ability, are prepared to listen and change, and also speak the truth as you see it, neither you nor others can expect more.

Self-doubt can develop when people challenge your perceptions and motives. It is important to listen to what they have to say – they may have things to teach you (although they may not be the exact things they imagine). But 'listening' does not mean uncritical adoption of other views. You need to subject their and your own views to scrutiny and to discuss the issues thoughtfully. This is reflective practice. It is dialectic. It is learning.

Striving to be an outgoing person helps. People appreciate those who bubble with positive energy, take the trouble to put themselves in the shoes of others and don't get too wrapped up in their own anxieties. Things are likely to work out well enough if you can maintain an adventurous spirit and see the silver linings around dark clouds.

Yet the world of integrated care is turbulent and unpredictable. You need a plan to recover balance when you wobble. You need a plan to maintain inner peace.

PAUSE: What do you do to maintain inner peace?

Three different ways of losing inner peace

You are likely to have your balance and inner peace threatened in three different ways:

1 **Losing your sense of self:** Your role requires you to dip in and out of many different stories. You will have many identities. You can become confused as to who you are in all of this, and in what ways you have been successful, or not. This is loss of balance in the sense of *losing your narrative unity* – losing a sense of a life story that is coherent and positive. You can regain and maintain this by reviewing how your past, present and anticipated future make sense as a whole story. Meditation, reminiscence, creative interaction with others, friends and psychological therapies can all help.

2 **Being uncertain about when and where to act:** Being effective in complex evolving situations is like windsurfing. Your actions need to consider changing wind direction, underwater currents, and your own strength and skill. You may feel that you have lost your ability to judge when to go with the wind and when to tack against it. This is loss of balance in the sense of *losing confidence in your vision*. you can regain and maintain confidence through strategic planning, mentors and organic metaphors.

3 **Becoming overwhelmed by the number of different things:** You work with large numbers of people, at different stages of development. You will support many different projects and at least one is likely to be in crisis at any time. This is loss of balance in the sense of *losing control*. You can regain and maintain control by managing information, using system maps, timelines and lists and activating your network of teams.

Things that help to maintain inner peace

Maintain inner peace by retaining narrative unity

Narrative unity means that people want to make their lives coherent as positive whole stories. This coherence does not mean endlessly repeating the same things. It means continually adapting and transforming to co-evolve with those who make us who we are. Because everything else is changing around us, it's as if we have to change to remain the same. It helps to ask: 'Who do I want to be in five years' time?' and 'What can I do now to travel in that general direction?'

We must remember that significant people in our life stories are part of us. We are part of them. Attempts to deny this or to control their versions of our shared story merely fragment us. We all find it difficult to look deep into a mirror and see ourselves as others do; and identify the things we need to change; and change them. But that is what we must do.

Life stories are continually evolving. We can reminisce about times gone by and enjoy the continuity of values and skills from then to now, but we can't become our old self exactly. Time and life experiences move us on, even if we don't want to. So we have to develop our life stories in ways that are faithful to the past, but also face forwards to become a new me/you/us. I need to continually transform myself to be the best me I can be.

Transformational change alters the way I think and act. It puts new mental models in my mind that lead me to think and act differently – perhaps to be more appreciative and less self-preoccupied. It challenges me to rewrite my account of my life to be less someone who hides away from the world and more someone who engages with it optimistically, creatively and wisely. Transformation involves the 'death' of an old me and the 'birth' of a new me.

Reflecting on real-life situations helps to bring to the surface the things I need to change to remain me. If I bring to mind an encounter or a story, it helps to ask these questions:

- What did I do to make it good? What did I do to make it less than good?
- What did the other person(s) do to make it good, or less than good?
- What does this say about how I think and how they think?
- Do I want to change? What precisely will I change?

Some of these reflections can be too painful to do alone. Counsellors and therapies help.

Techniques that allow anxieties to melt away and a smile to appear are important. Ways to go beyond words, where 'I can lose myself' are worth considering. Meditation, yoga and music can do this. Others use gardening, dancing and sport. Every spiritual and faith tradition has its methods. It is tempting to use whatever seems immediately attractive, but make sure that it has the power to go beyond the superficial. We each need to exhort ourselves: Be courageous. Be optimistic. Be the one you want to become.

Here are some things that help to prepare for inner transformation:

- **Use techniques that help you to be alive in the moment:** Mindfulness. Appreciate others. Meditation. Music. Mantras. Reconnect with my past and future.

- **Creatively interact with those who matter to you:** Play games. Touch. Laugh. Have fun. Make it feel good.
- **Do things that make you feel good:** Exercise. Play music. Dance. Paint. Go to the theatre. Appreciate beauty, cooking, children, elderly, gardening.

Maintain inner peace by retaining confidence in your vision

'Vision' means ideas about the world as well as sensory perceptions. Those who think in controlling, linear ways will not be able to see the non-linear connections that systems thinkers can see, so they will challenge and disbelieve you. Organic metaphors help to retain confidence in the connections you see between different things. Here are some examples:

- I am a *gardener* who enables interaction between insects, birds and flowers.
- I am a *conductor* of an orchestra who coordinates different musical inputs.
- I am a *surf-boarder* weaving in and out of towering waves.

Metaphors like these help to see what to do in real-life situations. They help to distinguish between things I *can* do, and things I can't. I should worry about the things that I can do, and not feel responsible for things that are beyond my control or ability.

Here are some things that help us to regain confidence in our personal visions:

- **Strategic planning:** Anticipate my future support needs using backwards mapping (Chapter 7). Appraise situations quickly using rapid appraisal (Chap 7).
- **Develop networks of high performing teams:** Develop my network of trusted individuals and teams, and invite them to give me honest feedback.
- **Images and phrases that keep me alive in the present:** Try out images and phrases that keep me vital. I can repeat them, like a mantra, to keep me – me.

Maintain inner peace by retaining control

Maintaining control in a complex, changing world means making sense of its various strands. Like a bus driver navigating bus routes, to feel in control I need information, routes and support to travel. I need to:

a) *Create information systems:*

- **Record and retrieve information,** e.g. about projects, events and organisations
- **Contacts who can provide information about new things,** including new approaches to integrated care, funding opportunities, and potential partners
- **Maintain administration support** for bulletins, marketing, events

b) *Create system maps, timelines and lists:*

- **Draw a system map(s) of integrated care in my area:** Leave it on the wall to help everyone to remember and critique
- **Have clear timelines:** Stages in the annual cycles of improvement; feedback of project teams; dates of meetings

- **Make lists of tasks:** And lists of lists. And colour-coded lists that link different lists of lists. And check that they genuinely ensure that things are done on time and in synchrony

c) *Nurture networks of teams*

- **Ongoing communication with teams:** A way to repeatedly communicate with individuals and teams who share my values and my life story
- **Instigate new projects that build from past ones:** It helps to re-enliven those teams that are particularly important to me; look out for opportunities to reunite them in new ways
- **Call for help:** Sometimes I just need help. I must remember to give back

Self-actualisation

Everything converges on the present. It is the only place where anyone can change anything. Here we make sense of the past and shape the future. The present moment is always there, but it is always in transition – always moving onto the next moment. It is not easy to be fully present in the present – the mind wanders. Being fully alive in the present requires high-level listening skills, appreciation of the richness of the surrounding world and presence of mind to draw back from issues that will unhelpfully suck you in. It is easy to be preoccupied with yesterday's mistakes and tomorrow's fears; less easy to refocus on the simple things you can do to make things better. Too many people spend too little time paying attention to the valuable things in front of them, and too much time defending themselves against imaginary enemies.

The skill of being alive in the moment is called *mindfulness*. Everyone needs mindfulness.

The skill of acting in effective and positive ways is called *self-actualisation*. Remaining effective in the midst of complexity may be the same thing as self-actualisation.

Maslow put self-actualisation at the top of his 'hierarchy of needs'. The term has been used by psychologists to mean realisation of full potential, expressing one's creativity, quest for spiritual enlightenment, pursuit of knowledge, self-discovery, self-reflection, self-realisation, self-exploration and the desire to give to others.

Goldstein believes that self-activation is the master motive, the only real motive: 'the basic drive'. Similarly, Rogers wrote of 'the curative force in psychotherapy – man's tendency to actualize himself, to become his potentialities . . . to express and activate all the capacities of the organism' (http://en.wikipedia.org/wiki/Self-actualization).

In the language of narrative unity, self-actualisation involves mental and emotional agility to move quickly between different parts of my life, checking that they make sense as a whole. It involves having the power and presence of mind to act in the present to be faithful to both past experiences and ambitions for the future.

Chaos theory makes much of the butterfly that flapped its wings and caused a hurricane the other side of the world. We tend to assume that the butterfly did not know what it was doing – it flapped by chance, and accidentally 'won the lottery'. Self-actualisation suggests that there are 'no such things as accidents' (apologies to Master Oogway in the Dreamworks film *Kung Fu Panda*). The butterfly *felt* the right time to flap the wings by being in tune with – integrated with – the world around it. It did not have a specific purpose in mind, but acted to synchronise with the 'winds of change' it felt.

Self-actualisation and internal balance might both include the following components, each of which can be practised and learned and developed at never-ending levels of sophistication:

Self-actualisation = Mindfulness + Narrative unity + Strategy + Appreciation + Practice

Travel hopefully

Leading integrated care, like self-actualisation, requires us to tune into positive patterns in the world that are invisible at first sight. To do this we need also to tune into the positive patterns within ourselves – listening to others and listening to ourselves is the same skill. We tune into them by listening with humility, learning with an open mind, participating with generosity and valuing the creative input of different perspectives.

Leading integrated care requires a vision for integration, and the will to do things that incrementally achieve it. It requires us to see things that help to transform what *is* into what *might be*. It gets easier with practice, but it is never easy. It requires *harmonising* more than control; *being* more than telling. There is no protocol to guarantee success. Instead we need to be guided by the aim to *travel hopefully*.

Exercise: devise a personal plan for self-actualisation

Part IV

Understanding community-oriented integrated care

In Part IV:

Who might find Part IV useful?

The image to support Part IV: A human face

Living systems have mechanistic and co-adaptive aspects

Medical training emphasises the mechanistic aspects of living systems

Implications of the image of a human face for community-oriented integrated care

Introduction to Part IV: community-oriented integrated care – a verb *and* a noun; a machine *and* a living organism

Box: Linear, emergent and transformational change

Chapter 13: The story of community-oriented integrated care. Community-oriented integrated care means that coordination of care and health improvements happens close to where people live. Care plans and local health communities help people to collaborate for shared care, self-care and healthy living.

Chapter 14: General practitioners are sense-makers. Primary care practitioners and managers see, more than others, different aspects of health and different contributions to care. Patients have multiple problems and the most important often lurk below the surface. To address these, practitioners think at several levels, repeatedly see people over time, bring hidden factors to the surface, and give patients things to think about and things to do.

Chapter 15: Health, identity and relationships. Health is being alive in the moment, able to reach out to, and positively interact with others, forming networks of relationships that define our identities. A healthy person rises above adversity to develop a coherent and positive life story – each person is the lead actor in the 'feature film' that is their life and co-actor in the 'films' of others. Health means that your life story is a story to be proud of. Health promotion encourages people to seize opportunities of the moment to make good things happen.

Chapter 16: Three paradigms of inquiry illuminate evolving stories. The success of laboratory (positivist) approaches to science has marginalised approaches that reveal hidden connections and emergent aspects of truth. They see control rather than harmony. The result is a mechanistic approach to healthcare that has difficulty in seeing the complex and evolving aspects of health. Guba has analysed three paradigms of inquiry that in combination can overcome this limitation.

Who might find Part IV useful?

This section is written for those who wish to understand a science of interconnectivity and transformation, including teachers and those who design, lead and research integrated care.

Part IV explores the history and potential of community-oriented integrated care (COIC), and the natural role of general practice/family medicine within it, particularly in the UK National Health Service (NHS). COIC is multidisciplinary, team-based care that operates close to where people live. It reminds us that health and care are everyone's responsibility. No one, however talented, can do it all on their own.

Integrating care and health promotion means seeing beyond structures of control, to also see systems that help people to harmonise their ways of working, and processes that bind them together with trusted relationships. This requires a better balance between 'laboratory' *positivist* science where individual particles cause change by directly impacting on other particles, and 'real-world' *constructivist* science where particles constantly change in response to other particles that are themselves constantly changing. This has been called a complex, adaptive, living system.

Part IV describes:

* **Health** as *positive narrative unity* and disease as challenge to that coherence
* **Development** as *cycles of inter-organisational learning and change*
* **Research** as *illumination* – what you see depends on how you look

Part V continues exploration of theory, to consider human interactions that develop trusted relationships within networks, organisations and systems.

The image to support Part IV: A human face

Look at a human face and you will see expected parts – bones, lips, eyes. You would be surprised if they were not there. Each part does what it is expected to and can often be repaired if broken, as though a machine component. Look again and you will see constantly changing expressions in response to internal and external stimulation – smiles, frowns, questions, listening, un-listening . . . And these can change second by second as the situation changes. This is not a machine; this is a dynamic, living system.

The entire human body has features of both a machine and a living system. *Machines* behave in predictable ways with clear, linear links in a chain of actions. *Living organisms* co-create things through multiple-way interactions that respond to, and shape, events.

Integrated care has both machine-like care pathways and living organism-like shared care. It is neither one nor the other, but both. If you look for machine-like behaviour, you will see it. If you look for living system behaviour, you will see that too.

Living systems have mechanistic *and* co-adaptive aspects

A science of interconnectivity has to reconcile an ages-old tension between things that are complete in themselves and do not change, and things that creatively adapt to things around them. The first is like a predetermined machine, the second a co-adaptive,

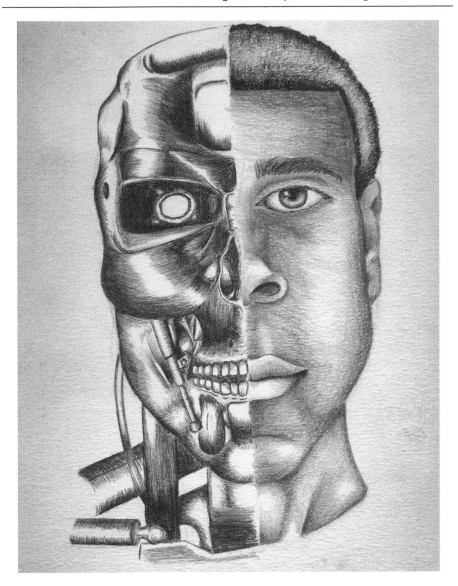

Figure IV A human face

living system. The different ways that machines and living systems behave has been described as a contrast between the *natural and social sciences*, the *science and art of medicine*, and *quantitative and qualitative* approaches to inquiry.

A central argument in this book is that everything has both mechanistic and co-adaptive aspects. Both are needed – they enable complementary things to happen. Even a living system has predictable, machine-like aspects. They are different paradigms so cannot be integrated in linear ways and you need different lenses to see them.

Authors from different disciples show that mechanistic and co-adaptive aspects can come together in different ways. Organisational behaviour theorist Karl Weick describes how leaders make sense of complex situations by considering both known and emerging truths. Physicist Fritjof Capra explains that the basic unit of life is a *cell*, and cells contain *particles* that are the basic units of a machine. Physician Robert Winston describes living synapses in the brain that grow in response to objective stimuli and from this change the ways people think and act. Biologist Candace Pert describes microscopic hormones that flood the body and feedback loops that allow the whole body to respond to complex stimuli.

Karl Weick

Weick attributes to Burns and Stalker (1961) a description of the fundamental differences between mechanistic and organic systems. Organic systems need things like 'shared beliefs about the common interests . . . and a quality of interaction' (p. 65). (See also Chapter 14.)

   Wieck, K. *Sensemaking in Organisations*. Thousand Oaks, CA: Sage, 1995

Fritjof Capra

Capra argues that the basic unit of life is not a particle but a cell, that is 'membrane bounded, self-generating, organisationally closed metabolic network(s)' (p.13). It is a living system, constantly re-creating itself and constantly exploring its surroundings. At any time, a snapshot will make it look static, but to understand how it works you have to see it in action.

   Capra, F. *The Hidden Connections*. London: Flamingo, 2003

Robert Winston

Living systems adapt in response to stimulation. Winston explains:

> The most important stage for brain development is the beginning of life, starting in the womb and then the first year of life. By the age of three, a child's brain has reached almost 90% of its adult size. This rapid brain growth and circuitry have been estimated at an astounding rate of 700–1000 synapse connections per second in this period. The experiences a baby has with her caregivers are crucial to this early wiring and pruning and enable millions and millions of new connections in the brain to be made. Repeated interactions and communication lead to pathways being laid down that help memories and relationships form and learning and logic to develop. This means a human baby's brain is both complicated and vulnerable . . .
>
> The new science of epigenetics is discovering more and more how our genes and our brains are affected by the lives we lead. For example, Champagne et al. showed that (related and unrelated) mice put in the care of loving mothers (who are attentive and lick them caringly) grow up to be better mothers themselves

when they have pups. This effect is so strong that it can even stretch over two generations, with granddaughter mice being better mothers and able to cope with stress better too, all because their grandmother took good care of their mother. These long-lasting benefits of good parenting in mice are dependent on chemical changes in the DNA of the mice.

 Winston, R. and Chicot, R. (2016) http://dx.doi.org/10.1080/17571472.2015.11 33012

Candace Pert

Pert has demonstrated that vast numbers of polypeptides are produced by the brain in response to internal and external stimuli. They flood the body with profound effects on other cells. These previously invisible particles are a main mechanism to keep the whole body integrated – and they do it through ongoing, dynamic, 'invisible' interactions.

This reveals a mechanism whereby the body and the mind connect. It explains the healing power of everyday things like a smile or a touch. It explains how people with 'negative energy' cause illnesses in themselves and in those they relate to. It explains how 'emotional exhaustion' happens when people encounter hostility and stress. Pert's 'molecules of emotion' bear comparison to the invisible radio waves from mobile phones that have an effect only when the sender and the receiver are on the same wavelength. Inside the body these molecules affect those cells that are receptive, providing instant whole system effects. Within integrated care these are the millions of friendly gestures that build a healthy community – invisible at a distance but very real when experienced.

 Pert, C. *Molecules of Emotion*. London: Simon & Schuster (Pocket Books), 1999

The new insight these authors bring is *play*. The connected parts do more than control and compete. They creatively interact and mutually co-adapt, often in unpredictable ways.

Medical training emphasises the mechanistic aspects of living systems

The human body is made up of cells that interact across their semi-permeable membranes. This is an example of Checkland's 'soft systems' – nutrients are exchanged according to the abilities of the cells involved and the opportunities of the moment. However, the human body also has 'hard systems' – the heart pumps blood one way around the cardiovascular system. The nervous system and the gastrointestinal system are similar.

 Checkland, P. *Systems Thinking, Systems Practice*. Chichester: Wiley, 1993

Medical student education emphasises the mechanistic aspects of the human body. This explains why doctors often emphasise a mechanistic image of life that readily sees facts but is less attuned to co-creativity.

Implications of the image of a human face for community-oriented integrated care

This image reminds us that integrated care is complex. Stripping out either mechanistic or organic aspects will destroy it, in the same way that stripping out the cardiovascular system or Pert's microscopic instruments of change will destroy a person. It is not enough for one discipline to consider mechanistic and another organic phenomena – everyone needs to consider ways to use both in the process of building the future from the issues of the present. Organisations like general practices and clusters of practices can be nurtured as cells within a body that is healthcare. Health care needs *both* linear systems (such as care pathways) *and* organic systems (such as trusted relationships developed from cycles of inter-organisational learning and change).

PAUSE: What images of integrated care do you use?

Introduction to Part IV: community-oriented integrated care – a verb *and* a noun; a machine *and* a living organism

Integrated care needs healthy organisations and systems as well as healthy individuals. It needs pathways to integration in the same way a town needs interconnected roads. Like a vibrant community, it needs to provide its members with a sequence of valuable things to do, and success stories that build confidence and motivate to do more.

A key message repeated throughout this book is that integrated care can be systematically developed, but not solely with the tools of laboratory science (termed *positivism*). Positivism imagines things to be separate *objects* that interact with each other in direct 'linear' ways. On its own it is unable to see the dynamic interactions between different objects that make them become integrated. These aspects can be seen with other theories of knowledge, termed *critical theory* and *constructivism*. All three sciences are needed in integrated care.

Integrated care and health promotion does have *object(ive)* features – staff, buildings, services, care pathways, diseases treated, for example. But these are not the things that make it vibrant and sustain; these require ongoing collaborative learning and coordinated change. Teams, organisations, communities and others become bound together through shared projects in which participants contribute to shared improvement projects. Integrated working is a dynamic ongoing process of positive human interaction. *If you want to sell integrated care, think of it as a noun. If you want to lead it, think of it as a verb.*

People often think of integrated care as a machine. They decide what each individual component should do, monitor standards to make sure that people do these things, then collapse the model every few years and replace it with the 'latest model'. This may be useful in a factory where individual operators undertake the same repeated tasks. But 'operators' of integrated care have to co-create personalised plans and multi-task in overlapping teams. These sophisticated team-tasks cannot be achieved through 'top-down' control, nor solely through the efforts of individuals, however talented.

When considering the treatment of diseases it is often helpful to think of integrated care as a machine full of hard-wired care pathways – a *hard mechanical system.*

When considering health improvements it is often better to think of integrated care as an organism full of harmonising, co-adapting cells – a *soft, living system*. The human body is an example of both. It is integrated and controlled not by top-down control nor bottom-up actions, but by non-stop inter-cellular co-adaptation and whole-body messaging. Yet within it, hard systems like the cardiovascular system are also essential. *If you want integrated care to treat diseases one at a time, think of it as a machine. If you want to create healthy communities think of it as a living organism.*

Linear, emergent and transformational change

Community-oriented integrated care and health-promotion needs whole-society transformation towards collaborative ways of working. Transformation is a participatory, co-creative activity, as is shown in the example of a nightclub in which a jazz band tries out a new style of music.

When a band improvises, one player takes the first step of a new musical pattern. The other players copy the notes. This is linear change – the same tune played by others. Then, at high speed, the players zoom back and forward in their minds to make sense of it, comparing patterns from past tunes and possible directions for the tune to go. One catches the tune and develops it, then throws it to someone else who plays with it. Those who are particularly 'in tune' are even able to improvise at the same time. At the end the whole band 'gets it' and plays at the same time to make a harmonious conclusion. The audience applauds. Everyone smiles. They go home with a determination to come back for more.

This is an example of emergent change because the new tune came out of interaction between those involved. It is an example of a transformational change because the whole system changed (the nightclub is now a jazz club). It is an example of health improvement because it gave the participants a good, coherent story to tell.

The jazz band example reveals useful insights into emergent and transformational change:

- *The players trusted each other to creatively respond.* If a musician tried something new and other team members ignored it, the creative move would stop.
- *They included linear steps as well as innovation.* Their 'new patterns' include old patterns, put together in innovative ways as well as things never heard before.
- *The experience binds them togther.* The prefix 'co' or 'com' signals this potential – it means 'jointly, with, together'. Players co-construct, co-design, co-develop, co-llaborate, com-bine, com-mit. Their actions bind them together as a comm-unity.
- *The players were chosen to provide complementary inputs.* The band did not form by chance; the players were of equivalent skill and had different instruments
- *The whole system was in the room.*

In this example the change *emerged* from the actions of the band; the response of the audience translated it into *whole-system transformation*. They all agreed – we like this music.

Now let us consider an example of transformational change on a bigger stage. The television cameras witness a football team co-create a new pattern of play – as innovative as the jazz band's new tune. Other teams try the pattern out and find that is good for them too. Soon everyone is doing it. The whole system of football transforms the way the game is played.

The examples show that transformational change requires ownership from all concerned. The football teams that copied the new pattern did not themselves create it, but they did make it their own. The jazz-band audience had nothing to do with the creation of the new tune, but it resonated with them; they felt a part of its creation, as a whole community.

The examples show that transformation does *not* need everyone to be in the same room at the same time, but it does need mechanisms for all members of a system to feel in some way related to what happened in the 'room'. It shows that *emergent change* can also be an *incremental transformation* – when there are mechanisms for people from all parts of the system to make it their own.

The story of community-oriented integrated care

Key message: Health-care systems throughout the world are moving towards community-oriented integrated care that emphasises team-working and local communities for health.

In this chapter:

- What is community-oriented integrated care?
- 2014 Commonwealth Fund Report
- Scientific inquiry is not the only thing that underpins medical practice
- Primary care coordinates care for people in their real-life contexts
- 1978 Alma Ata Declaration advocates partnerships for integrated working
- Need for general practice leadership of integrated care and health promotion
- Experiments in multidisciplinary teamwork and partnerships in general practice:

  o Public health practitioners and community groups
  o Universities and community-based organisations
  o Extended primary care teams

- Experiments in policy for integrated working:

  o Participatory research develops communities for health
  o Whole-system interventions support multiple-way partnerships
  o Community development agencies attempt integration at scale

- West London integrated care programme
- A new localism
- The present – integration *and* disintegration
- Relevance of COIC to the WHO vision of comprehensive primary health care

What is community-oriented integrated care?

If you think of organisations as living systems you pay attention to certain features such as connections, relationships, meaning. If you think of mechanical systems, you pay attention to design, control mechanisms and so on.

(Pratt et al., *Working Whole Systems*)

Integration means that different services and disciplines work in coordinated ways. Community-oriented integrated care (COIC) has features of *community-oriented primary care* (COPC) in that it combines health-promoting and disease-curing activities for general practice patients, families and communities. It differs by also enabling integration for health and care throughout local geographical areas (beyond individual practices), and aligning care pathways to those areas. COIC combines mechanical coordination with networks of high-performing teams. Coordination and teamwork matter because both care and health promotion improve when people work in synchrony. Localities matter because they provide *shared developmental spaces*, so different organisations can lead complementary things. Trusted relationships matter because people need trust to work creatively with each other, and produce effects more than the sum of the parts.

Integrated care is especially needed for people who have long-term, complex conditions; *care plans* help different people to contribute to *shared care* and *self-care*. *Integrated health promotion* is needed for whole-population participation in health improvements; clusters of general practices in geographic areas work with public health and many others to build healthy environments and healthy communities. Annual cycles of inter-organisational learning and change help people throughout the system to harmonise their ways of working.

This chapter describes the origins of COIC, and why primary care should lead its development in partnership with public health, universities and many others.

2014 Commonwealth Fund Report

The 2014 Commonwealth Fund Report reveals that the UK enjoys some of the best primary care in the world. When compared with ten developed countries it scored highest for quality, access and efficiency; and second highest for equity (behind Sweden). This is despite having the second lowest per capita spend (New Zealand was lower). Then, extraordinarily, in the category of 'healthy lives' it scored tenth – second only to the USA for poor outcomes.

The category of 'healthy lives' includes: 1) deaths that could have been prevented with timely and effective care; 2) infant mortality; and 3) healthy life expectancy. These things obviously cannot be improved by primary care on its own. They require many different organisations to align their efforts to promote health – public health, local authorities, schools, community groups, families and many others.

Primary and community care practitioners don't need the Commonwealth Fund to see the need for integrated working between different agencies at local, community level. Every time practitoners see a patient with a long-term condition or difficult life circumstances, or someone who is elderly or lonely, they recognise what's needed – families, friends, neighbours and other social support, getting meals on tables, keeping active, getting out of doors. It is obvious, surely, that sometimes people need a variety of help to do these things and take part in activities that put a smile on their faces – music, dance, photos, chats, gardening . . .

Scientific inquiry is not the only thing that underpins medical practice

The development of scientific method in the seventeenth century is often cited as the basis of modern medicine. The idea, attributed to Isaac Newton, that *causes* have predictable *effects* underpins the medical notion that diseases should be treated with *evidence-based medicine*. Actually, the idea that doctors should observe carefully the outcomes of treatments goes back much further than Newton. It was a basic teaching of Hippocrates in ancient Greece.

Ancient Greece had other less 'scientific' healing traditions that are also to be found in modern-day medical practice. The God of healing, Asclepius, prescribed rest in a place of peace – an approach we now advocate to recuperate from illness. Aristotle's four humours resemble modern-day advocacy of balance in all things. Ancient Greek emphasis on keeping clean, a good diet and exercise are standard modern-day public health exhortations. In reality modern doctors combine evidence-based treatments with a variety of 'non-medical' recipes for physical, social, mental and spiritual well-being.

The idea that doctors are a unified discipline that administers evidence-based treatments is relatively new. Julian Tudor Hart summarises the development of medical professionalism:

> Modern British medical professionalism developed during the first half of the 19th century, culminating in the medical act of 1858. . . . . The currently accepted model of what a good doctor is became developed early in the 20th century, when medicine began to make serious claims to association with science.
>
> (pp. 43, 44)

The unification of medical practice at the turn of the twentieth century coincided with heightened awareness of the effect of poverty and ill-education on health. The shocking state of health of the UK population was revealed when half of the recruits for the Boer War (1899–1902) were found to be unfit for military service. This led the 1906 Liberal government to introduce free schools meals, school medical services and health visitors. Public health practice entered a new phase – beyond sanitation to healthy public policy.

Of course the world then turned upside down – two World Wars were separated by the Great Depression. Naturally, when we are vulnerable it is easier to see that we need others. These vulnerability-creating events may have been what was needed for wholesale realisation that citizens in a healthy society must care for others as well as for themselves.

In 1942 the UK government set William Beveridge the task of discovering what kind of Britain people wanted to see after the war. He identified five 'giants on the road to reconstruction': poverty, diseases, ignorance, squalor, idleness. To defeat these, Beveridge proposed social security, a national health service, free education, council housing and full employment.

Post-war action on Beveridge's plan can be seen as the beginning of community-oriented integrated care – a serious attempt to align the efforts of different disciplines to develop healthy, empowered citizens and communities. Disciplines *were* aligned, but in a structural, 'vertical' way, without mechanisms to integrate 'horizontally' between them. So each developed its approach to public service in relative isolation from each other, and with only scant understanding of each other's roles.

The work was carved up into different specialities – doctors were 'body mechanics'; public health practitioners dealt with 'rats and drains'; the State provided jobs; schools taught children how to think. And the Church did the touchy-feely bits. They had no reason to work more closely.

In any case each discipline needed to get its own house in order; GPs too. The National Health Service (NHS) began on 5 July 1948. Two months later, 93 per cent of the population was registered with a GP. At that stage GPs were isolated, uni-disciplinary, solo, mostly male medical practitioners who had no preparation for the coordinating role about to be put onto them, and without resources to do anything other than 'firefight'.

Primary care coordinates care for people in their real-life contexts

General practice as it is known today bears little resemblance to the surgeon-apothecaries of 1858 and the isolated general practitioners of 1948, except that they all see people in their real-life contexts – 'warts and all'. GPs witness 'real life', every day. They see the effects on health of a mish-mash of things – relationships, poverty, education and a sense of meaning, as well as diseases. They see families and communities as well as individuals.

Modern general practice has a pivotal coordinating role in health care, both locally and throughout the system. It is no longer isolated and no longer uni-disciplinary. Extended multi-disciplinary primary care teams treat patients with a full range of illnesses, including severe mental, social, spiritual and physical diseases. People present with a combination of depression *and* social isolation *and* poor internal balance, as well as with asthma, bedbugs, cancer, diabetes and other letters of the medical alphabet. Real life doesn't come in neatly carved-up disease categories. Real life is an integrated mix of everything. We need integrated care and integrated health promotion because life itself is already integrated.

To be adequate to the way that *people* present, rather than how specialists carve up the work, GPs need skills beyond the management of specific diseases. Generalists, more than specialists, need to see more of the whole context of a person's health and illness. They need to see whole systems of care and contribute to whole systems of health promotion. This broad role was argued by pioneer GPs. These pioneers shaped the founding values of the UK College of General Practitioners that was established in 1952 and received its Royal Charter as the Royal College of General Practitioners (RCGP) in 1967.

John Horder, before he became president of the RCGP, co-founded the 1974 Leeuwenhorst European Study Group that created a consensus about the general practice/family medicine role that became accepted throughout Europe and is recognisable today. This states that general practice/family medicine:

- 'Makes efficient use of health care resources through co-ordinating care, working with other professionals in the primary care setting, and by managing the interface with other specialities, taking an advocacy role for the patient when needed. This coordinating role is a key feature of the cost effectiveness of good quality primary care.'
- 'Develops a person-centred approach, orientated to the individual, his/her family, and their community. Family medicine deals with people and their problems in the context of their life circumstances, not with impersonal pathology or "cases".'

By the late 1970s, there was widespread agreement that general practice should promote health as well as treat diseases, as witnessed by the 1977 book *Trends in General Practice*:

About child care: 'Services provided for children by general practitioners include not only traditional medical care, but also psycho-social care of a child within a family group [and] a team approach with nurses and health visitors attached to the practices.'

About the elderly: 'The role the general practitioner as the co-ordinator of health care for the elderly is certain to become a dominant part of future general practice.'

About fertility and family medicine: 'the family doctor [needs to be] an informed advisor in questions of family fertility . . . [aware of] associations between poverty, ill health and large families . . . and concerned with family size, family spacing and the prevention of unwanted pregnancies.'

 Fry, J. (ed.) *Trends in General Practice*. London: RCGP, 1977

1978 Alma Ata Declaration advocates partnerships for integrated working

It all came together in September 1978 at the international conference at Alma Ata. 134 member states of the World Health Organization (WHO) and 16 international organisations reached a consensus about 'Health for All by the Year 2000'. This meant whole-system integration – in the horizontal direction between community-based organisations for the health of local populations, and in the vertical direction between generalist and specialist medical workers for disease care.

 Okoro, C. Primary health care in London: onwards from Alma Ata, *LJPC*, 2008, 1: 61–65

It was then called *comprehensive primary health care*. This includes all contributions to health and care. John Macdonald identified its three essential 'pillars' – *participation, inter-sectoral collaboration* and *equity* – in his book that he aptly subtitled 'medicine in its place'.

 Macdonald, J. *Primary Health Care: medicine in its place*. London: Earthscan, 1992

The Alma Ata Declaration identified *primary health care* to be *the* key way to realise its vision for integration, but this meant much more than 'primary care' as we know it today. Declaration VII states: 'Primary health care . . . involves, in addition to the health sector, all related sectors and aspects of national and community development, in particular agriculture, animal husbandry, food, industry, education, housing, public works, communications and other sectors; and demands the coordinated efforts of those sectors.'

Need for general practice leadership of integrated care and health promotion

Ever since Alma Ata, countries throughout the world have pursued policies for general practice leadership of integrated working. The term 'primary care' emerged to mean multidisciplinary general practice teams. The UK announced a 'primary care-led NHS'.

Primary care is a good place to lead integrated care because the closer you get to where people live their everyday lives the more you can see the large number of factors that impact on their health. Further away, as in specialist arenas such as hospitals, conversations naturally revolve reason for being there – usually their diseases.

Primary care also has all the raw ingredients. It has highly motivated, intelligent practitioners and managers who on a daily basis encounter the complexities of health and idiosyncrasies of people. It includes a broad range of clinicians – core GP teams and extended primary care teams that include a range of allied health professionals.

Primary care practitioners also work regularly with practitioners from every part of the system, the A–Z of the medical, social and mental health dictionaries. So they are uniquely well placed to see how multiple dis-eases interact within a person and how multiple practitioners interact within a whole system – and how to improve both.

This isn't often called 'integration'. It is usually called 'good general practice'.

Experiments in multidisciplinary teamwork and partnerships in general practice

The 1978 Alma Ata Declaration led to broad awareness of the potential of general practice to lead comprehensive primary health care. Health promotion, collaboration and community development were emphasised. Team-working became a watchword – core GP teams, extended primary care teams, local organising teams, shared leadership teams.

Many initiatives witnessed the excitement stimulated by Alma Ata. Many initiatives did not involve general practice at all. For example, Michael Money brought together 20 examples of health improvements arising from non-medical groups and communities.

 Money, M. (ed.). *Health & Community: holism in practice*. Dartington: Green Books Ltd, 1993

Other initiatives *did* involve general practice, in particular partnerships between general practice and public health, general practice and universities, and between different members of extended primary care teams.

Partnerships between general practice, public health and community groups

Reminiscent of the 1930s Peckham Experiment, Kark's *Community-Oriented Primary Health Care* (COPC) included community diagnosis, health surveillance and focused projects to improve the health of vulnerable groups (e.g. mothers and children). His book gives case studies of general practices in urban Israel and rural South Africa that developed COPC.

Kark, S.L. *Community-Oriented Primary Health Care*. London: Appleton-Century-Crofts, 1981

Liverpool, UK, developed a *Healthy City 2000 Project* that worked with Ashton and Seymour's concept of the 'new public health'. It formed a strategic coalition of organisations to support health promotion, community development and broad-visioned primary care.

 Ashton, J. and Seymour, H. *The New Public Health*. Buckingham: Open University Press, 1988

Tudor Hart established a research and teaching general practice in Glyncorrwg, a South Wales village with a population of 5,000. Here he combined general practice and public health roles, using data about health need to set up projects to address these needs.

 Hart, J.T. *A New Kind of Doctor*. London: Merlin Press, 1988

Partnerships between general practice, universities and community-based organisations

Many partnerships between universities and general practices developed in the 1980s and early 1990s in the UK. One was Teamcare Valleys. The University of Wales College of Medicine worked with 2,000 primary care practitioners from 156 general practices and their associated organisations (e.g. Family Health Service Authorities and community services) to develop communication, education, field projects, and practical support and advice.

 Bryar, R. Teamcare Valleys: a multifaceted approach to teambuilding in primary health care. Chapter 5 in Pearson, P. and Spencer, M. (eds) *Promoting Teamwork in Primary Care: a research based approach*. London: Arnold, 1997, pp. 56–68.

Extended primary care teams

In the 1980s, the term *primary care* emerged, to mean multidisciplinary general practice teams. Extended primary care teams formed – core GP teams worked closely with named practitioners from health-authority employed *community services* including district nurses, health visitors and allied health professionals.

The *Association of General Practice in Urban Deprived Areas* (AGUDA) became a network of general practices who explored new ways to work with local communities and with extended primary care teams. AGUDA retained its reputation as a forward-thinking network through annual conferences held in different UK cities and hosted by local general practices, often in collaboration with health authorities and non-governmental organisations.

The *National Primary Care Facilitation Programme*, based in Oxford, became an umbrella for a huge number of primary care innovations. It initially focused on training facilitators to undertake audits and develop well man clinics in general practices. As different towns and cities developed their own models of integrated working, it became a forum for discussion of the broader principles of primary care facilitation and cross-pollination of ideas. Here are some of many models that were discussed to identify transferable lessons:

- Liverpool's *local multidisciplinary facilitation teams.* Four teams of locally employed practitioners were trained to facilitate collaborative working and improvement projects in general practices within localities (geographic areas of 70,000 population). They worked hand in glove with many other strategic initiatives including audit in general practice and the Liverpool Healthy City 2000 project.

 Thomas, P. and Graver, L. The Liverpool intervention to promote teamwork in general practice: an action research approach. Chapter 13 in Pearson, P. and Spencer, M. (eds) *Promoting Teamwork in Primary Care: a research based approach.* London: Arnold, 1997, pp. 174–191

- Sheffield's *Towards Coordinated Practice.* A facilitation team supported GPs practices to collaborate with each other and evaluate improvement projects.
- South London's *Camberwell Project.* Through a 'hub and spoke' arrangement, lead general practices linked with the local university to help practices to innovate and share learning

The Health Education Authority *team-building workshop programme* built multidisciplinary primary care teams and strategic infrastructure at the same time. Five general practice teams of 5–12 individuals of different disciplines attended a three day residential workshop where they designed a practice service. An inter-organisational *Local Organising Team* facilitated the workshops to develop a network of leadership between their institutions.

 Spratley, J. *Joint Planning for the Development and Management of Disease Prevention and Health Promotion Strategies in Primary Care.* London: Health Education Authority, 1991

Experiments in policy for integrated working

In 1979, only a year after the Alma Ata Declaration, WHO policy abruptly shifted away from comprehensive primary health care with its emphasis on building communities for health, towards targeted interventions like breast feeding, immunisations and family planning.

The reason for this change has been attributed to a disbelief that the broader vision was realistic. It also conflicted with UK/US policy of the time that came to be called the 'new public management' – or more crudely 'markets and targets'. This policy was suspicious of 'bottom-up' developments that had indirect and subtle effects on culture. It preferred 'top-down' control with 'line management'. Language of change in the NHS became dominated by market-inspired terms like consumers, efficiency and the purchaser–provider split.

By the mid-1990s in the NHS the emphasis on building communities for health had been replaced by targeted initiatives like GP Fundholding (from 1991), and projects that were evaluated as stand-alone entities. The image of integrated care as a *machine* was strong in this phase.

Many good things happened. For example, care pathways for stroke care showed how to quickly transfer patients from the street to specialised medical care, and the National Institute for Clinical Excellence (NICE) provided evidence to grass-roots clinicians of the effect of different kinds of treatment. On the other hand, this phase witnessed increasing medical specialisation and 'marketization' of health care, inhibiting the growth of generalism, integration and multidisciplinary team working.

The Blair government of 1997–2007 tempered this emphasis on efficiency and accountability with 'third-way' socialism that valued community development as well as thoughtful planning for whole society health. Primary care groups (1999) gave way to primary care trusts (2000) with GP input. Blair's mantra 'education, education, education' allowed a re-entry of the language of *learning organisations* into polite planning circles.

In 2008 the Director-General of WHO urged a return to comprehensive primary health care (see Introduction) – 'more important than ever' to address contemporary health issues.

Many things became clear through these initiatives, including:

- **Integration is not simple:** If you use a targeted approach, you often *reduce* integration by neglecting things you are not focused on. If you use a community development approach, progress is slow, evaluation is difficult and success depends on the skills of the leaders. In both it is easy to meander without achieving things of lasting value.
- **Integrated care needs both community development and targeted initiatives at the same time:** Community development projects need targeted initiatives to act on the problems they discover. Targeted initiatives discover (often too late) that to sustain improvements or act on insights they have generated, they needed to have earlier engaged the whole community concerned (e.g. the community of medical practitioners).
- **Integrated care needs long-term facilitative infrastructure** to support ongoing inter-organisational improvements, develop relationships in many directions, build communities, and increase the capacity of the whole system to act in integrated ways.
- **The science of whole-system integration is unfamiliar:** Weaving together multiple perspectives requires co-adaptation. Particularly valuable insights of how to achieve this come from *organisational learning* and *participatory action research* – people feel that they belong together when they inquire into their situation together, learn from this and take collective action to improve the situation – cycles of learning and change.

Many initiatives helped to understand the science of whole-system integration.

Participatory Research develops communities for health

De Koning and Martin described initiatives in India, Uganda, Bangladesh, Zimbabwe and Bolivia that enabled people to appraise their own situations and collectively improve them. They show that participatory approaches to inquiry help to build communities for health.

De Koning, K. and Martin, M. (eds) *Participatory Research in Health*. London: Zed Books, 1996

Whole-system interventions support multiple-way partnerships

The King's Fund piloted models of whole system integration in UK cities. Using methodologies of Future Search, Open Space and Real-Time Strategic Change (described in Chapter 10), they enabled people from many different sectors to co-design integrated systems of care. These provide evaluated models that can be strategically used to build networks and communities for community-oriented integrated care.

 Pratt, J., Gordon, P. and Plamping, D. *Working Whole Systems: putting theory into practice in organisations*. London: The King's Fund; 1999

Community development agencies attempt integration at scale

Mead's 31-country study of primary care innovation revealed six ideal types of primary care organisation: outreach franchise; reformed polyclinic; extended general practice; district health system; managed care enterprise; community development agency.

Of these, the *community development agency* most obviously develops communities for health, beyond medical care. He examined case studies in Peru, Costa Rica, Venezuela and Bolivia, in which they maintained 'health is a citizen, not a profession issue' (p. 100).

 Meads, G. *Primary Care in the Twenty-First Century: an international perspective*. Abingdon: Radcliffe, 2006

Further analysis of Mead's work revealed that his six ideal types naturally cluster into three models of different kinds of integration:

Model 1: Outreach franchise and polyclinic – integrating through medical practice
Model 2: Extended general practices and district health systems – integrating through multidisciplinary teams
Model 3: Managed care and community development agencies – integrating through networks, communities and systems

 Thomas, P., Meads, G., Moustafa, A., Nazareth, I. and Stange, K. Combined horizontal and vertical integration of care: a goal of practice-based commissioning. *Quality in Primary Care*, 2008, 16: 425–432

West London integrated care programme

The 2012 UK Health and Social Care Act led to clinical commissioning groups (CCGs) with strong GP leadership. This led to a renewed emphasis on GP leadership of health-care developments. The *integrated care pilot* in west London (population of about two million) helped eight Primary Care Trusts to create 50 localities of 50,000 population (at the time they were becoming clinical commissioning groups). In these localities, general practitioners met every month with colleagues from acute medicine, mental health and social services to devise care plans for those patients who might benefit from multi-agency input. New stages of this initiative from 2015 (as the *Integrated Care Programme*) included locality-based collaboration for integrated services and locally led innovation.

A new localism

By 2014, in the UK as with other countries, the increasing numbers of people with multiple long-term conditions had made large numbers of people aware that centralised models of health care are inefficient, as patients go from one specialist to another along parallel care pathways, duplicating effort and often missing the bigger picture of someone's health. This led to a renewed emphasis on multidisciplinary primary care teams that create care plans for patients with complex conditions. The pendulum started to swing again towards locally oriented integration, that became called 'new localism'.

 Ferlie, E. (2010) Public management 'reform' narratives and the changing organisation of primary care, *London Journal of Primary Care*, 3: 2, 76–80, DOI:10.1080/17571472.2010.11493306

In planning circles, the hunt for the *best* model of integrated care began to give way to discussions about how to discern what models could usefully be adapted to specific situations. There developed broad acceptance that good human relationships and mechanical efficiency are both needed; 'bottom-up' and 'top-down' approaches to change are both needed; horizontal and vertical integration of care are both needed.

Following the lead from Canada, in 2012 UK cities started to cluster general practices into localities of 30–50,000 population, called 'health networks' when addressing medical concerns, and 'local health communities' when addressing broader health issues.

There were also attempts to bring closer together the functions of provision and purchasing and to facilitate collaboration at local levels. In 2014, GP Federations – coalitions of GPs (as providers) – aligned to the same areas as clinical commissioning groups (GPs as commissioners) and local authorities. In the same year, general practices were funded to create care plans for 2 per cent of their practice population most likely to need hospital admission.

Renewed awareness of the strategic importance of general practice is witnessed in the 2014 *Five Year Forward View*. It states: 'The foundation of NHS care will remain list-based primary care . . . GP-led Clinical Commissioning Groups will have the option of more control over the wider NHS budget, enabling a shift in investment from acute to primary and community services.' *Integration* was widely considered the solution to the NHS problems. A nation-wide set of 50 'vanguard' sites was set up in 2015 as a 'blueprint for the future of NHS and care services'. They are presently evaluating five types of 'new care models', which could support community-based coordinating hubs, needed for integrated working:

1   Integrated primary and acute care systems (PACS) – joining up GP, hospital, community and mental health services

2   Multi-speciality community providers (MCP) – moving specialist care out of hospitals into the community
3   Enhancing health in care homes – offering older people better, joined up health, care and rehabilitation services
4   Urgent and emergency care – new approaches to improve the coordination of services and reduce pressure on A&E departments
5   Acute care collaborations – linking hospitals together to improve their clinical and financial viability

 New care models – supporting the design and implementation of new care models in the NHS. www.england.nhs.uk/ourwork/new-care-models/ (accessed 19 January 2017)

The present – integration *and* disintegration

It seems wrong to applaud the shift towards integration in UK health policy without acknowledging other policy shifts towards dis-integration. At the time of writing (March 2017), the UK population has narrowly voted to leave the European Union – separating from an alliance that has enabled a period of unparalleled peace and prosperity throughout Europe. At the same time, Scotland is moving towards a referendum to split from the United Kingdom. At the same time, the UK's strong ally the United States has narrowly voted for a president who seems to think only in linear, controlling ways.

On the face of it, popular desire for short-term concrete, linear control has defeated desire for more longer-term collaboration and harmony. On the face of it.

One danger of this shift towards linear, compartmentalised thinking is the development of a culture of individualism and short-termism that will not accept the social values of shared care, the complexity of integrating processes, and the long-term and diffuse outcomes of integrated working. One opportunity, or challenge, is to describe these values, processes and outcomes in ways that make sense to those who think in compartmentalised ways.

The need to describe dynamic, evolutionary processes in concrete terms is not a new one. There will always be a need to explain complex things in ways that fit with what people want to see. This is the rationale for 'Third Way' politics. As long as political discourse is framed as combat between opposites, change means a lurch from one side of the 'boat' to another, making everyone 'sea-sick'. 'Third Way' politics combines deep strategy for sustainability with appealing 'sound-bites' (p. 155) that satisfy specific desires, including 'right-wing' desire for heirarchical control and 'left-wing' desire for social justice (pp. 40–41).

 Giddens, A. *The Third Way: the renewal of social democracy*. Oxford: Polity Press in association with Blackwell Publishers Ltd, 1998

UK new care models is a 'Third Way' idea. It is a set of inter-linked packages of integration. Each package contains complex interactions. Each is valuable in its own right; in synchrony they might have the power to facilitate whole-system collaboration and social justice, while including mechanisms of control. Routinely gathered data can evaluate, in real time, the combined effects on cost and quality of these inter-linked packages, including effects on well-being, citizenship and capacity, as well as economics.

Local debate about data, combined with personal experience and pilot improvement projects, increases understanding of how to sustain progress and helps to shape thoughtful, locally relevant approaches to thorny issues like self-care and public–private partnerships. This might appeal to the 'right' by ensuring cost-effectiveness and control. It might appeal to the 'left' because it advances participatory democracy and emancipation.

The stage is set for a grand experiment of what it is to be a liberal democracy in the modern world. All might agree that integration is desirable but structural approaches are too bureaucratic. All might agree that other approaches are needed. One test-bed is health care – case studies of integrated working.

Case studies should describe their plans to build relationships across multiple boundaries, and link these initiatives to stimulate a broad sense of 'we'. This 'we' must value harmony between people of different backgrounds as well as negotiated control. At local level these might be called *communities for health*. In other contexts they might be called *networks of leadership teams* that facilitate mutual understanding and collaborative action, and link 'big pictures' to self-interest.

Other public services, for example schools, should also become case studies, each with their own plan to achieve 'added extra' through inter-linked packages of integrated working.

If this seems a strange idea, try this even stranger one – GPs should lead this. Given their lack of training, preoccupation with focused medical problems and being already overwhelmed, this might seem impossible to consider. But it has logic:

- GPs are intellectually able – 'A+' science students so good at solving complicated puzzles. GPs are often altruistic – they choose to apply their skills to improve health. GPs work with the breadth of human experience. GPs experience on a daily basis glitches in all parts of the system, the complexity and potential of the human condition, the centrality of relationships to health, and the enormous number of factors that contribute to well-being and dis-ease.
- GPs have many potential partners to share the work with. There are different languages and histories of course, but all public services aim for healthy individuals and healthy societies – public health, schools, social services, police, and so on. Then there are faith groups, political parties, voluntary groups, charities, and so on. At present many are struggling to apply to a modern context their traditional values. Many are ready for transformational steps in partnership with like-minded partners.
- In the UK at least, policy already aims to achieve a grand alliance for health and care, with GPs in the lead. This is the goal of the 2016 Sustainability and Transformation Plans and New Care Models. The 2016 *GP Forward View* furthers this with ambitious plans for investment, recruitment, workload and infrastructure to enable success.

So GP leadership of community-oriented integrated care is already happening – as an evolutionary response to the practical difficulties of health-care organisation. This organic process in health care could be re-badged as an example of what it means to be a low-bureaucracy, high-quality twenty-first-century liberal democracy.

Making a success of integration in health care, at scale, requires us to answer three difficult questions:

1   What reforms to the GP role will make it fit to lead community-oriented integrated care?
2   What definition of health will unite people to collaborate for healthy societies?
3   What approach to knowledge generation and change is adequate for this?

I explore these questions in the remaining chapters of this part. The implications for policy and action are explored in the final part (V).

Relevance of COIC to the WHO vision of comprehensive primary health care

Community-oriented integrated care (COIC) is a way to practically link the idea that *health is a medical thing* with the idea that *health is a citizen thing* – to make treatment of diseases relevant to the experience of health. It includes shared care for people who are sick, health promotion that helps people to help themselves and local communities for health. A healthy citizen is one who is ready, willing and able to act not only for their own health but also for the health of the people around them; and indeed for the health of the planet. This is not merely altruism. It is enlightened self-interest as people come to recognise that their fates are tied up with those of their neighbours.

COIC is a slogan, an appealing sound-bite intended to translate to the modern context the founding principles of the NHS. It is a response to Margaret Chan's call, described in the Introduction, to create community-based coordinated hubs with the power to re-enable comprehensive primary health care.

COIC requires a new mind-set about health-care organisation. Health *services* are set within health *systems*. Initiatives improve the health of individuals, families and communities at the same time, as well as treat diseases. Infrastructure supports shared leadership in both vertical and horizontal directions. Vertically, care pathways ensure good medical care. Horizontally, inter-disciplinary collaboration develops communities and networks for health and care. Everyone contributes to environments for health, self-care and care for others.

To achieve COIC, coalitions of general practices need to work within geographic areas in collaboration with social care, voluntary care, public health, schools, business and many others. Together they will build local health communities through annual cycles of locality-based learning and change, using methods that help people to work well with others. GP Federations and clinical commissioning groups will oversee this, working with hospitals, out-of-hours services, academics, professional bodies and politicians.

Many things need to be worked out:

1   Which organisation(s) and disciplines should lead which aspects? What models facilitate ongoing, multiple-way collaboration for what constituencies in what contexts? What approaches to leadership development work best in what situations? What evaluation markers help to monitor improvements in well-being, citizenship and capacity, as well as economics?

2   The science of COIC needs to be understood and taught at every level – from early parenthood to end of life care. It needs to be in the core school curriculum. You don't 'own' COIC. Instead, you constantly re-create it through collaborative action – like a running stream it becomes stagnant if you stop the flow of energy. Approaches to research, development and leadership that are adequate for this multi-faceted and constantly evolving entity are discussed in Chapter 16.

3   If health is more than a set of diseases, what is this thing *health*? This is discussed in Chapter 15.

4   The expectation that GPs can lead this alone is unrealistic. And for that matter, how do they deal with the A–Z of medical, social and mental illnesses and health promotion anyway? This is the subject of Chapter 14.

Chapter 14

General practitioners are sense-makers

Key message: Community-oriented integrated care needs high-quality general practice.

In this chapter:

- A general practitioner (GP) consultation
    - is a complex event
    - is a snapshot of a story-in-evolution
    - includes specialist expertise
- Three functions of general practice
- GPs help people to write better stories
- A GP – jack of all trades and master of sense-making
- Community-oriented integrated care needs shared sense-making
- Integrating three different consulting styles in primary care practice
- Daytime, emergency and out-of-hours primary care can all support integrated care
- Different ways for patients to interact with primary care practitioners
    - Services within general practices
    - Services shared between general practices
    - Community services that relate to general practices
    - Social services that relate to general practices
    - Specialist medical services that relate to general practices
- Strategic dilemma – finding what you need when you need it
- Strategic dilemma – building trust
- Relevance of general practice to community-oriented integrated care

A GP consultation is a complex event

Medical students are taught that a patient visiting their GP brings a 'presenting complaint' – a single problem to be solved. The GP analyses the problem using a structured sequence of questions and actions, takes a history, examines the patient and arranges tests. The GP solves the problem by making a diagnosis that may require medical treatment and advice.

This is a very useful approach on the rare occasions when a patient presents with a single delineated medical problem.

The trouble is that even patients who present with a single problem usually have an intertwined mish-mash of dis-eases. Indeed, the most important issues often lurk below the surface, invisible even to the patients themselves. So to really improve someone's health a GP needs to provide opportunities, over time, for a patient to recognise these multiple issues and do something about them, with the support of various agencies. Those words, 'over time', are really important.

A GP consultation is a snapshot of a story-in-evolution

A GPs usually has a 'surgery' of ten-minute appointments. In that time the GP reviews the past notes, calls the patient from the waiting room, takes a history, examines the patient, forms a plan, says goodbye and writes up the notes.

Often there are many problems, often very complicated problems. To deal with these, experienced GPs use the ten minutes efficiently. They think at several levels at the same time. They recognise complex patterns of illness and health. They exclude 'red flags'. They surface hidden factors. They ask questions that make the patient reflect and feel that they 'own' the emerging plan. They write notes that make it easy to pick up the story next time.

A consultation is rarely the only event. And conducting a consultation in a linear fashion is rarely helpful. This is because a consultation is part of a process that the textbooks don't really describe at all. A consultation is one of a sequence of encounters. Those encounters include overlapping conversations continued by different members of the primary care team.

A GP consultation includes specialist expertise

When a GP doesn't know the answer, he or she seeks help, there and then, or before the next consultation. Typically, GPs use local guidelines, colleagues, emails and telephone advice lines to support their decision-making. This is how these 'jack of all trades' are able to master the A–Z of the medical, surgical, social and mental health dictionaries.

Three functions of general practice

In *A Flourishing Practice?* Peter Toon presents his analysis of the role of general practice. He concludes that general practice has three functions:

1   Biomedical treatments to relieve suffering and cure disease
2   To prevent disease
3   To help patients construct a flourishing narrative

He describes this third function as the 'heart of practice' – 'the main purpose of medicine is to help patients construct a flourishing narrative' (p. 45). This is a hugely important point. He's saying that general practice has a mission beyond treating and preventing diseases, and that is to help people find health, and to do so by constructing a 'flourishing narrative'.

 Toon, P.D. *A Flourishing Practice?* London: RCGP, 2014

GPs help people to write better stories

An experienced GP rarely follows Toon's three functions in a rigid way. He or she skips from one aspect to another in a free-flowing conversation. The conversation can take many different forms and depends on the individual clinician, the individual patient and the issues of immediate concern. It can involve musing aloud the non-linear patterns she/he is noticing, planting ideas, inviting reflections and making leaps of intuition. Here are some examples:

> Interesting, you have come every June for the past three years about a similar thing; I wonder what that might mean?

> I know you are worried about your daughter who you brought today; you know I am not that worried about her – but I am a bit worried about you; are you OK? You look a bit pale.

> How's school? . . . How's your wife? . . . How are things generally?

> Sometimes when you get a flurry of things going wrong it is life telling you that you need to do a 360 per cent review – where you are going, your social life, your routines.

These questions help to explore what a flourishing narrative might mean for that particular person. Here the GP is facilitating learning; which is what the word 'doctor' means – *teacher*.

A GP – jack of all trades and master of sense-making

John Launer describes 'narrative-based primary care' as a consultation style that helps patients to achieve a flourishing narrative. Rather than drill down to one complaint, the clinician follows the little 'asides' that people make as they describe their story:

'It [headache, depression, pain] started when I was at work . . .' – '*What is your job?*'
'I had just had lunch with a colleague . . .' – '*Oh, who was that?*'

And by following these little asides, a GP can bring to the surface a range of associated factors inside which may lie more fundamental explanations for why someone feels unwell.

This is *active* listening, where you intrude on someone's flow of ideas with timely reminders that you are listening at a deep level. It resembles an everyday conversation more than a forensic analysis. Problems *are* analysed, but in a way that allows connections between various factors to be revealed. It shifts attention away from diagnosing delineated diseases towards making sense of the more complex, non-linear patterns in someone's life story.

So Launer echoes Toon by saying: 'The job of a general practitioner is to help people to write better stories.'

 Launer, J. *Narrative-Based Primary Care: a practical guide*. Abingdon: Radcliffe Medical Press, 2002

A narrative style helps to make sense of complexity. Instead of asking a patient to list their problems, a GP asks a patient to describe what has happened since they last felt well, like a video unfolding. This reveals non-linear associations between factors that are invisible in a simple list. It can reveal the way that people think about how things happen, what Argyris and Schon call 'theories in use' – hidden mental models that drive people's behaviours.

Surfacing the way someone thinks reveals something of their 'life script' – their sense of who they are. For example a person may think of himself or herself as a defensive victim or fighter or loner – not flourishing. Changing something so deep is *transformational*. Launer and Toon challenge us to surface and challenge these script in general practice consultations. We must routinely oscillate between superficial and deep reflections, and so stimulate deep reflections in patients that might help them to incrementally transform their life stories.

It is not just life transformations that benefit from a fuller understanding of someone's story. It also helps when diagnosing and treating illness. Consider two people with identical severe headache, both developed yesterday. A narrative approach reveals that the first person had been well until recently; the second had been overworking for years and had often experienced such headaches at times of stress. Their different stories direct our attention in different ways. Even when they have the same 'diagnosis', revealing more of the context helps to consider the best course of action, including non-standard treatments.

Here are some everyday examples where GPs routinely deviate from standard treatment of an illness because it makes sense in the light of the broader story:

- The person whose immunity is low, whether from chronic illness or stress, is more at risk from infections than others, and should be treated earlier and more aggressively.
- The person with asthma who gets a viral infection should automatically increase their asthma medication.
- The person at the end of their life who develops a chest infection might benefit from a family conference about whether or not to treat the infection.

Community-oriented integrated care needs shared sense-making

There is a science to sense-making, described most eloquently by Karl Weick. Being able to tell a coherent story about how various strands of my past make sense as a whole powerfully affects what I do in the future. Weick argues that sense-making is more than *interpretation* because it involves *authoring as well as interpretation, creation as well as discovery* (p. 8). Sense-making looks both forwards and backwards, co-constructing ideas, metaphors and scenarios that link what is known with what is not. Weick quotes Schon about how sense-making involves complexity, co-creativity, certainty and uncertainty:

> When professionals consider what road to build, they deal usually with a complex and ill-defined situation in which geographic, topological, financial, economic and political issues are all mixed up together. Once they have somehow decided what road to build and go on to consider how best to build it, they may have a problem

they can solve by the application of available techniques, but when the road they have built leads unexpectedly to the destruction of a neighbourhood, they may find themselves again in a situation of uncertainty.

(p. 9)

Weick quotes Thayer that leaders are facilitators of sense-making, or 'sense-givers':

A leader at work is one who gives others a different sense of the meaning of that which they do by recreating it in a different form . . . in the same way that a painter or sculptor or poet gives those who follow a different way of 'seeing' . . . the leader is a sense-giver.

(pp. 9–10)

Sense-making provides a framework to conceptualise and explore the world:

Sensemaking involves placing stimuli into some kind of framework. That enables them to comprehend, understand, explain, attribute, extrapolate and predict . . . [it is] grounded in both individual and social activity . . . When people make sense of things they read into [them] the meanings they wish to see; they vest objects, utterances, actions and so forth with subjective meaning which helps make the world intelligible to themselves.

(pp. 4, 6, 14)

Shared sense-making creates 'glue' that binds people together:

The glue of organisational culture is usually portrayed as 'shared meaning' . . . Although people may not share meaning, they do share experience . . . actions, activities, moments of conversation, and joint tasks, each of which they then make sense of using categories that are more idiosyncratic. If people have similar experiences but label them differently, then the experience of shared meaning is more complicated than we suspect. If people want to share meaning they need to talk about their shared experience in close proximity to its occurrence and hammer out a way to encode it and talk about it . . . they need to see their joint saying about the experience to learn what they jointly think happened.

(p. 188)

 Weick, K. *Sensemaking in Organisations*. Thousand Oaks, CA Sage, 1995

If GPs are to take a lead role in integrated working, they need to be sense-makers. They need to facilitate cycles of learning and change (Chapter 19) that help others to make sense of things by 'hammering out' ways to describe shared, integrated stories. They need to build interlinked opportunities for people from different parts of the system to makes sense of the whole system and from this devise coordinated strategy. Parts I–III describe models that do this in practical everyday ways.

Chapter 15 explores further the link between sense-making, health and identity. This chapter continues by describing roles, functions and disciplines in primary care that need to be included in this grand process of sense-making.

Integrating three different consulting styles in primary care practice

Responding to patient problems is one of three types of consultation in general practice. The others are planned care (care plans for long-term conditions) and emergency care (when things have to be done in a hurry). Each type involves a different consulting style:

- **Responsive care:** works thoughtfully from the presenting complaint to reveal other issues that might be relevant (e.g. other diseases; emotional and social issues)
- **Planned care:** follows the care plan goals, using protocols and patient data
- **Emergency care:** focuses on the immediate threat, e.g. accidents, stroke, appendicitis, acute mental illness, child abuse

Primary care clinicians, including GPs need to switch effortlessly between these styles. They might spot the need for emergency or planned care when someone presents with something quite different – for example, he/she may notice a skin cancer or the need for a care plan for someone who presents with a common cold.

Daytime, emergency and out-of-hours primary care can all support integrated care

Different types of primary care are more or less suited to different roles in integrated care:

- **Daytime general practice** sees all aspects of health and illness. So having a central role in orchestrating care plans and system integration makes sense.
- **Unscheduled care centres** tend to see people who have accidents and acute illness. Their main role should be as a place for accident avoidance, self-help for minor illness and signposting other self-care resources.
- **Out-of-hours services** tend to see people who have exacerbations of long-term conditions. It therefore makes sense for them to contribute to care plan updates.

Different ways for patients to interact with primary care practitioners

There are many ways to interact with primary care other than a face-to-face GP consultation. Telephone consultations, home visits and a variety of clinics are obvious ways. Less obvious are letters, leaflets and the practice website that support self-care. Patients can see various members of the extended primary care team. They can heed the advice in their care plans. Primary care should also help patients to become experts in their long-term conditions, so they can self-monitor (e.g. monitor their own blood pressure or blood sugar) and self-care (e.g. alter doses of medication when appropriate). This reminds us that the aim of accessing primary care expertise is less to be 'treated' and more to have trustworthy information to make good decisions and to be comfortable with those decisions.

Primary care is much more than general practice. It is a network of community-based teams, some employed by general practices and some by other organisations. Community-oriented integrated care requires these teams to reinforce each other's roles. Leaflets and podcasts designed by one type of practitioner are used by others and directly by patients. For example, a practice nurse might give out a leaflet on welfare rights; a counsellor might provide a list of family-planning services; the practice website signposts parenting videos.

The following services are often available in UK primary care.

Services within general practices

General practice clinics:

- Diabetes, and other long-term conditions
- Teleconferencing with specialists, for example dermatology
- Counselling
- Well man and heart health
- Well woman and contraception
- Well baby and Immunisations
- Exercise, yoga, complementary therapies
- Mental well-being and parenting
- Welfare rights

Services shared between general practices

Collaboration between neighbouring general practices often happens for:

- Out-of-hours cover
- Advice from *GPs with special interest* (e.g. diabetes, palliative care)
- Care for long-term conditions (e.g. diabetes) and specific techniques – minor surgery, contraceptive devices and ring pessaries, acupuncture, osteopathy, warfarin initiation

Community services that relate to general practices

GPs relate to community services provided by trusts and independent organisations:

- Community nurses and palliative care nurses
- Health visitors and school nurses
- Physiotherapists and rehabilitation teams
- Foot care specialists, dieticians, occupational therapists
- Mental health and well-being practitioners
- Speech and language therapists
- Rehabilitation
- Continence service
- Respiratory service (including lung function teats)
- Tissue viability and leg ulcer service

- Learning disability services
- Substance abuse

Social services that relate to general practices

GPs relate to a range of social services provided by local authorities and voluntary groups:

- Carers
- Meals on wheels
- Child and adult safeguarding
- Translating services
- Home adaptations
- Occupational therapists
- Transport
- Drop-in centres and day care
- Residential care
- Child care and after school clubs
- Sports and recreation facilities

Specialist medical services that relate to general practices

GPs relate to a huge number of specialist medical services provided by hospitals and others:

- Intermediate care specialities (e.g. obstetrics, diabetes, musculoskeletal)
- Medical specialities (e.g. respiratory, renal, neurology)
- Surgical specialities (e.g. ophthalmic, cardiac, cancer)
- Mental health specialities (e.g. psychiatrists, counsellors, family therapy)

Strategic dilemma – finding what you need when you need it

The number and scope of services is so big it can be really difficult simply knowing where everyone is. So it's vital that information on services is continually updated and referral processes follow a familiar pattern that is easy to understand – referrals, advice lines, feedback on episodes of care, data on overall performance, and so on.

Both clinicians and patients need to be able to navigate the whole system easily, and also contribute to improvements.

Strategic dilemma – building trust

As well as knowing where people and services are, trusted relationships and team-working are essential for good quality. Integrated care needs the vast numbers of practitioners in all parts of the system to develop a shared sense of identity, so that 'we' really know who "we" are. Everyone needs to work in synchrony. Everyone needs to be a team player.

This means more than just knowing who's involved. It requires regular opportunities to develop relationships across disciplinary boundaries.

Relationships between disciplines can be built when discussing patient care. But the scale of relationships to be built makes it unrealistic to do it entirely opportunistically or solely from a practice base. Comprehensive coordination needs a geographic locality where different organisations repeatedly communicate for patient care and strategic developments. To make this easier, since 2012 general practices in the UK have been clustering into geographic areas to build *health networks* and *local health communities*.

Relevance of general practice to community-oriented integrated care

General practice sits at the place in the health service where everything connects. Primary care practitioners see all aspects of health and care. They regularly see glitches in the whole system. That's one reason why primary care teams need to contribute strongly to the *practice* of community-oriented integrated care.

The pivotal position of primary care coupled with its powerful political voice means that it should also have a strong role in *leading* community-oriented integrated care. Practitioners and managers need *public health skills* to assess health need and promote health for whole populations. They need *applied research skills* to design and evaluate whole system improvement projects. They need *organisational development skills* to build relationships throughout whole systems of care. Partnerships with public health, academics and managers can bring in expertise. COIC requires all primary care practitioners and managers to have a basic grasp of these skills.

This has profound implications for the skills learned by health-care practitioners and managers, both in their formative training and through ongoing learning:

1   Everyone in primary care needs to be a skilled *team player,* not just a team member. Like actors on a stage, team players are skilled at joining different teams at a moment's notice, even with people they barely know. They know how to make valuable contributions to different teams for shared care and for health improvements. In the future, primary care practitioners also need to contribute to shared leadership teams for integrating activities. This needs to go beyond their core teams and practices to broker strategic partnerships – with public health and local organisations to support a whole locality/whole population approach to health; with intermediate care clinicians to maintain high-quality care pathways for specific illnesses; with patients and community groups to enable self-care. How to interact with others as a good team player is discussed in Chapter 18.

2   Primary care practitioners and managers need to be skilled *action learners* and *systems-thinkers* – able to visualise links in a whole system, think at several levels at the same time and recognise complex patterns of illness and health. They need to be able to learn from and with colleagues and patients and others, as life-long, life-wide learners, for whom learning and reflection is a way of life. These are skills of a *learning organisation,* described in Chapter 19.

3   Primary care practitioners and managers need to be skilled at *leading participatory action research.* They need to know how to access information when they need it, including performance and health data, and decision support. They need to be

skilled at generating and combining different types of knowledge (Chapters 11 and 16) and engaging others in this, through seasons of activity (Chapter 3).

4   Primary care practitioners need to *understand health as well as illness*. They need to know that the mission of general practice is to help people to develop a flourishing narrative for health as well as to treat diseases. To do this they need to know what health *is*, rather than merely agreeing that it is more that disease. 'What is health?' is the subject of Chapter 15.

5   Practitioners of all kinds need to write up patient encounters as stories, rather than disconnected facts. This should reveal the multiple factors that interact when living life forwards, quite different from the retrospective justification of events as seen with hindsight.

6   Primary care researchers, developers and authors should use multi-method inquiry to generate knowledge and multi-media ways to describe what happened and what they have learned.

It is not only primary care practitioners and managers who need to be skilled at these things. For COIC to work in a way that helps to achieve comprehensive primary health care, all citizens need these skills and the ability to apply them at all stages of life. These are core skills that need to be re-learned at all educational levels, from primary school to tertiary education. Chapters 4 and 20 explore the implications for the training of health-care professionals, managers and everyday citizens.

Health, identity and relationships

Key message: We need positive, holistic understandings of health, identity and relationships.

In this chapter:

- Health is:
    - o the foundation for achievement
    - o a positive narrative unity
    - o rising above adversity
    - o feeling and acting as equals
    - o travelling hopefully

- Healthy individuals and healthy organisations:
    - o revitalise relationships
    - o move forward with incremental transformations
    - o use metaphors that have both machine and organic aspects

- We oscillate between 'I–Thou' and 'I–It' thinking:
    - o to integrate complex things
    - o to live life forwards
    - o to learn and change

- Becoming locked in 'I–It' thinking prevents healthy forward movement
- Words are co-constructed to give voice to experience
- Bird-nesting belief systems explain the need for incremental transformations
- Narrative unity shows how to promote health in complex situations
- Relevance of narrative unity to community-oriented integrated care

Health is the foundation for achievement

Often when people use the word 'health' they mean disease – part of the body has become faulty, making someone feel dis-eased. But health is a positive thing. A healthy person is alert to possibilities, creatively interacts with others, has adventures and laughs. Being healthy means being *alive* in the moment and able to make a difference to others. Health goes beyond words. It is often only recognised with hindsight – after you have achieved something you did not think you were capable of. Health is much more than disease.

Seedhouse describes health as the 'foundation for achievement'. This definition helps to focus attention away from the static 'state' of health towards the dynamic things people do with it. If I am an athlete, I require different combinations of physical, mental, spiritual and social health than if I am a shopkeeper. I need different levels of health if I am old or young, beginning or ending my life's work, dependent on others or have others dependent on me.

 Seedhouse, D. *Health: the foundations for achievement.* Chichester: Wiley, 1986

Health means fitting well within my life story – literally 'fit-ness'. The contextual nature of health explains the 1978 World Health Organization definition – 'Health is a state of complete physical, mental and social well-being and not merely the absence of disease or infirmity'. This does not mean a state of perfection but a state of physical, mental, social and spiritual health adequate for the things I have to do, or want to do, now and in the future.

Many words support this forward-looking understanding of health – well-being, happiness, flourishing, resilience, vision, action competence, and so on. But to live life forwards in a positive way an individual also has to integrate these forward movements with their past life story. To an individual, health means making sense of your life story as a positive whole.

Health is a positive narrative unity

Alastair MacIntyre presents a theory that helps to see health as a coherent and positive life story. He calls it 'narrative unity'. He argues that our identities are revealed in stories. This means that each person is the lead actor in the 'feature film' that is his or her life story, and a supporting actor in the 'films' of others. Health means that these are more than simply coherent – they must also be positive stories; stories to be proud of.

 MacIntyre, A. *After Virtue: a study in moral theory.* Second edition. London: Duckworth, 1985

A coherent life story gives someone an integrated sense of self. With it they feel confident. Without it they feel they are 'falling apart'. This reveals itself as anxiety. Symptoms of anxiety, for example fear of uncertainty, often arise from a dis-integrated life story – one in which bad things have not been overcome, or life transitions not fully completed. Beneath the surface often lurk past hurts and regrets, present pressures, or daunting future challenges. Anxiety can often be improved by rewriting the life script in a more positive way.

Social psychologist Eric Berne explains that 'life scripts' are initially formed in childhood and to keep them vital they are repeatedly modified in response to life experiences. He wrote: 'Each person decides in early childhood how he will live and how he will die, and that plan, which he carries in his head, is called his script' (p. 31).

These scripts may be based on illusions and can change in response to crises: 'Scripts are usually based on childhood illusions which may persist throughout a whole life-time; but [in some] these illusions dissolve one by one, leading to the various life crises described by Erikson' (p. 28). Scripts can change in response to life experiences from which someone learns: 'The destiny of every human being is decided by what goes on inside his skull when he is confronted with what goes on outside his skull' (p. 31). But such transformation is not guaranteed to happen: 'In most cases he has spent his life deceiving the world, and usually himself as well' (p. 31).

 Berne, E. *What Do You Do After You Say Hello? The psychology of human destiny*. London: Corgi, 1972

Berne makes the startling conclusion that *in most cases* people's actions are guided by illusions carried over from earlier in their life, especially childhood. Most of the time adults are replaying stories from the past, and *projecting* them onto others as though they are true now. They are *not* alive in the present. They are living in their past.

When illusions give someone a coherent life story that does not harm anyone, the deception may not matter. What does matter is that the life story casts the person as a *positive* actor who feels alive and active in the world, able to live life forwards optimistically. A life of abuse from birth to death is coherent, but would hardly be called *healthy*. Nevertheless, the abused person might consider him/herself to be healthy if he or she did not think or behave like a victim and was able to make good things happen. A healthy person thinks positively about him/herself and does positive things. He or she rises above adversity.

Health is rising above adversity

Erik Erikson (1902–1994) was a developmental psychologist and psychoanalyst known for his theory on psychosocial development of human beings. He coined the term *identity crisis*. His research with troubled children led him to propose eight life stages (in his final book he described a ninth – old age). Each stage challenges an individual to develop a skill needed for his/her identity to be healthy. If successful, they advance to the next stage with confidence. If not, they are left with a *basic conflict* that comes from not knowing if they can master the stage. To master each stage they must overcome the challenge in a positive way – a way that 'supports growth and expansion, offers goals, celebrates self-respect and commitment of the very finest' (p. 106). Recognising that they have the inner strength to make the more demanding *positive* choice is the liberating factor that allows them to overcome that *life crisis* and think of themselves as an integrated, healthy person.

 Erikson, E H. *The Life Cycle Completed*. New York: Norton, 1998.

Erikson's eight life stages are:

1   Infancy (birth to 18 months):

  • Basic conflict: trust vs. mistrust
  • Important events: feeding
  • Outcome: Children develop a sense of trust when caregivers provide reliability, care, and affection. A lack of this will lead to mistrust.

2   Early childhood (2 to 3 years):

  • Basic conflict: autonomy vs. shame and doubt
  • Important events: toilet training

- Outcome: Children need to develop a sense of personal control over physical skills and a sense of independence. Success leads to feelings of autonomy, failure results in feelings of shame and doubt.

3   Preschool (3 to 5 years):
- Basic conflict: initiative vs. guilt
- Important events: exploration
- Outcome: Children need to begin asserting control and power over the environment. Success in this stage leads to a sense of purpose. Children who try to exert too much power experience disapproval, resulting in a sense of guilt.

4   School age (6 to 11 years):
- Basic conflict: industry vs. inferiority
- Important events: school
- Outcome: Children need to cope with new social and academic demands. Success leads to a sense of competence, while failure results in feelings of inferiority.

5   Adolescence (12 to 18 years):
- Basic conflict: identity vs. role confusion
- Important events: social relationships
- Outcome: Teens need to develop a confident sense of personal identity. Success leads to an ability to stay true to yourself without needing to control others, while failure leads to anxiety and defensive/aggressive tendencies.

6   Young adulthood (19 to 40 years):
- Basic conflict: intimacy vs. isolation
- Important events: relationships
- Outcome: Young adults need to form intimate, loving relationships. Success leads to trust and mutuality, while failure results in loneliness and isolation.

7   Middle adulthood (40 to 65 years):
- Basic conflict: generativity vs. stagnation
- Important events: work and parenthood
- Outcome: Adults need to create or nurture things that will outlast them, often by having children or creating a positive change that benefits other people. Success leads to feelings of usefulness and accomplishment, while failure results in shallow involvement in the world.

8   Maturity (65 to death):
- Basic conflict: ego integrity vs. despair
- Important events: reflection on life
- Outcome: Older adults need to look back on life and feel a sense of fulfilment. Success at this stage leads to feelings of wisdom, while failure results in regret, bitterness, and despair.

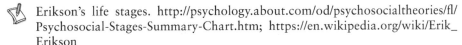 Erikson's life stages. http://psychology.about.com/od/psychosocialtheories/fl/Psychosocial-Stages-Summary-Chart.htm; https://en.wikipedia.org/wiki/Erik_Erikson

Health is feeling and acting as equals

The significance of Erikson's theory to *health* is obvious – a healthy person has mastered these stages. You are able to trust others (when they are trustworthy); you are autonomous (but also a team player); you are capable of initiative and industry; you have a confident sense of identity and are capable of intimacy. You live life forwards with confidence and responsibility, able to reflect, learn and change, appreciate others and work creatively with them. In contrast, you will be unhealthy when your thoughts are dominated by mistrust, doubt, guilt, inferiority, role confusion, isolation, stagnation or despair – these make you feel fragmented inside. A sense of internal fragmentation leads to contradictory ideas and actions – you may think of yourself as a victim, yet oppress others; you may constantly seek reassurance from others, yet reject those who could help you the most.

You need to have mastered Erikson's stages to interact with others as an equal – in ways that can build positive, mutually appreciative, trusted relationships and healthy communities. An integrated world cannot work if *most* adults lack trust, autonomy, initiative, industry, identity, ability to be intimate and creative. Society must help children to pass these stages successfully. Also, we must help those adults who need to belatedly catch up.

Not all children learn about positive, trusted relationships. In 2013 the UK National Society for the Protection of Cruelty to Children documented that one in five children experiences severe abuse. Even well cared for children may lack role models of good adult relationships – 50 per cent of marriages end in divorce and 30 per cent of children live with a single parent. Then there are children with learning, sensory or communication difficulties, children who are being bullied or groomed, children who have seen things or hold secrets that their minds can't deal with. Even the best parents may not know what their children need to learn. How to be team players and builders of healthy communities are not on the school curriculum.

There are children who never learn how to play 'good games' (Chapter 18) and from an early age become skilled at manipulating others. Some have to be adults before their time, as carers, interpreters and heads of households where the adults are not able. There are children who spend too much time on their own with computer screens for company, playing violent games that distort their understanding of a caring relationship. How can we expect them to be good team players and community developers?

More advantaged pupils can also be poor team players and community builders. They can accumulate a lot of facts without knowing how to apply their knowledge to facilitate healthy change. They will rightly feel good about being top of the class, but being 'top' encourages superiority rather than equality as a main goal. Some, perhaps many, will be on this so-called 'spectrum' where they, more than most, struggle to see things beyond their own cocoon of knowing. Later they go to university, and some go into medicine and become general practitioners, from where, decades later, they are expected to lead integrated care – often without the most basic grounding in how to integrate anything.

The challenge to think, feel and act as equal to others does not end in childhood. Even when Erikson's healthy attributes (trust, autonomy, etc.) are mastered as a child, later life provides plenty of opportunities to go backwards. Everyone encounters things that challenge their sense of self – rejection, loss, stress of one kind or another.

People who are able to retain a positive and coherent sense of their life story are more able to withstand life's stresses. This is Antonovsky's view. He developed his *Salutogenesis* theory (meaning 'source of health') from his observation that not all individuals have negative emotional reactions to stress. Some people, some Holocaust survivors, achieve positive emotional outcomes despite having had experiences that we might expect would break them completely.

Wikipedia explains how Antonovsky came to his views:

> In 1979, Antonovsky described influences that [influence] how people survive . . . in the face of even the most punishing life-stress experiences. In his 1987 book, he [described] that 29% of the women who had survived concentration camps had positive emotional health and were not emotionally impaired by the stress.

 Antonovsky, A. *Health, Stress and Coping*. San Francisco, CA: Jossey-Bass, 1979

Antonovsky, A. *Unravelling The Mystery of Health: how people manage stress and stay well*. San Francisco, CA: Jossey-Bass, 1987

Health is travelling hopefully

The emphasis made by Antonovsky, Erikson and Berne on overcoming adversity reminds us that good health is an active thing. Health means more than lying back and reminiscing a coherent and positive life story of my past. It also means developing my story into the future by interacting positively in the world. This means adventuring into the unknown, outside of my 'comfort zone', learning from my life's journey in ways that allow me to continually develop my sense of having a positive, coherent life story. Health means *travelling hopefully*.

Merely repeating the same rehearsed actions is not healthy – my life story will not develop. But neither is careless risk-taking – my life story might fragment. This challenges me to distinguish between risks worth taking and those that aren't. It challenges me to create *safe environments* that reduce risk. It challenges me to be alert to opportunities to share risk with others. I need to be prepared to receive and give support from and to others. I need to be *self-actualised* – ready, willing and able to adventure, learn and change.

Healthy individuals adventure in ways that enhance themselves and also enhance their fellow travellers. This mutuality is the source of trust in teams, communities, life partnerships, groups, organisations, networks, and so on. As well as developing trust, mutuality is the source of meaning, because a shared journey develops a shared story, and with this shared identities. And when strong ties develop it is often called *love* – a sense of being at one with other(s), separate yet bound together at the same time. Equal but different. Intertwined.

Healthy relationships are not static; they continually develop in ways that make those involved feel more than they can be on their own. Both in partnerships and in communities, relationships become unhealthy when controlled by one voice, or when those involved fail to communicate, or when they separate into different silos. In healthy relationships the individuals continue to creatively adapt to each other.

From a distance, a community looks like 'boids' – birds flocking. From a distance the flock looks like an integrated machine, each 'bird' doing what it is supposed to do. Look closer and you will see thousands of micro-adjustments that subtly alter the collective direction. This complex co-adaptation is how we move forwards as groups as well as individuals.

At any moment, I am a 'bird' faced with three options of how to think and behave:

1 Go wherever I want and risk breaking with the flock.
2 Follow particular birds within the flock, copying their actions.
3 Be mindful of the movements around me and flap my wings in ways that contribute to movement of the flock in new directions.

It is tempting to think of these not as options but as personality types, roles or ages – the 'parent' always does what they want; the 'child' always follows the lead of others; the 'adult' always adapts to others. Chapter 18 uses transactional analysis to show that reality is much more dynamic. People of all ages and roles continually move between 'ego states' of parent, adult and child to interact with others. This is how we move forward our life stories.

Chapter 16 uses the language of paradigms of inquiry to describe these three options as different ways of seeing the world and different ways of evaluating what happens as a result of an intervention. Each sees different aspects of the world.

This chapter continues by describing a need to repeatedly move between different ways of thinking, seeing and behaving to incrementally transform ourselves and our relationships.

Healthy individuals and healthy organisations revitalise relationships

As Taylor points out, we construct our sense of identity through interaction with others.

 Taylor, C. *Sources of the Self: the making of the modern identity*. Cambridge: Cambridge University Press, 1989 (pp. 509–510)

Through shared adventures we develop a shared story. This is how relationships develop. The words 'relationship' and 'relate' come for the same linguistic root – Latin *relatus*, to tell a story again. A relationship is a shared story, and it arises from shared adventures. It binds people together. It turns 'I' into 'we'. When someone you share a story with dies, a part of you dies too. When they succeed, a part of you succeeds too.

Shared stories connect people. They create *ties* that remain as long as the story matters to those involved. Once established, ties act as channels for people to affect each other – strengthening or weakening the relationship. Broadly speaking, actions that strengthen a tie contain positive attributes – trust, appreciation and energising spirit. Actions that weaken a tie contain distrust, rejection and distortion of truth. Strong ties make you *resilient*. This means that you will bend against pressure without breaking, and bounce back like a reed in the wind or one of Antonovsky's Holocaust survivors. Weak ties lack this empowering potential.

Just like individuals, partnerships and organisations need strong ties to be resilient – networks of creative, mutually enhancing, equal relationships. This resilience helps you to try out different things – to adventure. Just like individuals, these help them to become *established*. Just as with individuals, many partnerships and organisations, when established, stop building equal relationships and become controlling (without realising that they are harming themselves). This explains why 50 per cent of marriages end in divorce; when the excitement of the initial adventure is over it is easy to start to treat each other as objects to be owned rather than human beings to play with.

Here is a lesson for integrated care. To retain relationships we need to continually re-vitalise them. That is why we so often use the prefix 're' (meaning 'again') when talking about re-lationships. We re-discover ourselves by re-freshing them, by re-miniscing with our friends, and re-conciling hurts from the past. As well as having new adventures into the future.

But people often don't re-vitalise their relationships and they don't adventure. Perhaps they don't know how, or forget, or don't care, or are too frightened to try. It takes effort. It is much easier to stay in your 'shell', your 'ivory tower', your 'silo', where you can distance yourself from others, or try to control them. This is how we slide into poor performance and poor health.

A common reason for staying inside your shell is lack of resilience. We fear that if we come out we will not be strong enough to deal with what we encounter.

Here is a catch. We need strong ties to be resilient so we can adventure, yet we feel unable to create strong ties because we lack resilience. So we don't bother to have adventures.

Resolving this paradox requires transformation – we need to change from being defensive or fearful or introverted or accusing to develop the habit of routinely reaching out a hand of friendship.

Easier said than done. Transformation is not easy.

Healthy individuals and healthy organisations move forward with incremental transformations

> No man ever steps in the same river twice, for it's not the same river and he's not the same man.
>
> (Heraclitus)

Heraclitus reminds us that everything is changing all the time. For people who are skilled at engaging with the world, transformation is simply aligning with natural forces.

Berne and Erikson (above) explain that to be healthy, people need to repeatedly transform their 'life scripts' to meet the challenges of different life stages – adolescence for example. *Maturity* entails continually becoming a new me, by adapting to changes around me while also retaining a life story that is positive and integrated. This requires me to embrace new experiences without losing a sense of coherence of my whole life story. Transformation may be the 'death' of the 'old me' and the 'birth' of a 'new me', but the new me still values the old me. The butterfly values its previous life as a caterpillar, but feels no urge to go back to it.

Changing health care from silo-operating to integrated working requires a comparable transformation. A common *change narrative* is revolutionary – you shake everyone up at the same time with a 'big bang' intervention that collapses the entire system and puts another in its place. This approach can be effective – after all, it was the Second World War that led to the UK National Health Service in the first place. On the other hand, it has disadvantages – it loses experienced staff, organisational memory and things that are working well.

What is often forgotten is that mini-transformations happen all the time without the drama of adolescence and war, as we adapt to everyday life events. In fact it is *the* natural process of growth. As Heraclitus said: the only thing that is constant is change.

A healthy person does more than *change* in response to external change. He or she *learns and changes*, signalling that change does not have to be a passive, imposed thing. It can empower. It can be a resilience-creating experience. The healthy person changes as a positive choice. He or she analyses the situation, considers various options and chooses those that retain their personal integrity and also address the new external realities.

There is another change narrative in health care that has the potential to inform a less revolutionary and more evolutionary route to transformation – *continuous quality improvement*. This is usually interpreted as a sequence of stand-alone projects that do not link. By setting such projects within cycles of inter-organisational learning and coordinated change, they can enable a sequence of synchronised mini-transformation that can, in time, transform a whole system. This is the approach advocated here.

The organisational behaviour literature points to evidence that a series of synchronised mini-transformations might be a winning approach. McNulty and Ferlie describe a 1992–1997 intervention in a UK hospital to improve performance. It aimed for dramatic short-term improvements. At great cost, it used *business process reengineering* to stimulate 50–70 reengineering projects for six care processes (e.g. 'patient visits' and 'patient testing'). It focused on changing processes of patient care within established domains, so it lacked mechanisms for people from different domains to co-develop the whole system and to build on these year-on-year. The intervention failed to achieve expectations, causing its leaders to conclude that their original philosophy of a 'big bang' transformation was misguided, and a 'more incremental and evolutionary change philosophy' would have been preferable.

 McNulty, T. and Ferlie, E. *Reengineering Health Care: the complexities of organisational transformation.* Oxford: Oxford University Press, 2002 (pp. 124–130)

Healthy individuals and healthy organisations use metaphors that have both machine and organic aspects

> The only certainty in this life is change, but . . . that change can be directed toward a constructive end.
>
> (Henry A. Wallace)

Wallace reminds us that timely, thoughtful actions can alter the kind of transformations that happen. Different methodologies for transformational change make different assumptions about how the world behaves, and this leads to different kinds of actions.

For example, *business process engineering* imagines integrated care to behave like a *machine* – it therefore expects transformation to come from streamlining patient pathways. In contrast, *experienced-based co-design* imagines integrated care to behave like a *living organism* – it therefore expects transformation to come from mutual co-adaptations. Different methods will smuggle in complementary aspects that make them more hybrid than they appear at first sight. Nevertheless, the dominant metaphor powerfully affects expectations.

The person who has most highlighted the power of metaphor when facilitating change is Gareth Morgan. Morgan describes how the machine metaphor gives rise to controlling types of organisation like a bureaucracy – good when things are simple and stable. The living organism metaphor gives rise to *open systems* organisation like a learning organisation – good when things are complex and constantly changing. Each metaphor leads to different ways of thinking about how organisations behave, and different conclusions about policy.

 Morgan, M. *Images of Organization*. Thousand Oaks, CA: Sage, 1997

Metaphors that have both machine and living organism aspects help us to explore future uncertainty while still valuing past structures. Useful metaphors show how to creatively play between hard certainty and uncertain emergence; for example, the 'bite of skis on a snow', 'battling with the wind in a yacht' and 'surfing the waves'.

The metaphor of swimming in a river is like this. Going with or against the flow are both likely to be unsuccessful compared with working cleverly with the currents. You can learn to swim better, build a boat and use a buoyancy aid, for example. Grabbing hold of every piece of bank you come across will only bruise you and prevent you from advancing your journey. Instead the Buddhist metaphor of 'entering the water and making no ripples' is appropriate – you work *with rather than against* the multiple forces.

Capra likens the distinction between mechanistic and organic metaphors to Western and Eastern thinking. Western philosophy is combative – medical science shows how to kill bacteria and cut out cancers. In contrast, helping a body to help itself is more Eastern in philosophy. Of course we need both. That is why they are called 'complementary' rather than 'alternative'. They are good together: control *and* harmony.

 Capra, F. *The Tao of Physics*. Boston: Shambhala, 1991

Transformation changes a whole system – the direction of a whole river. A 'Western' mindset changes the direction of a river with mechanical diggers. An 'Eastern' mindset changes the direction of a river by integrating the efforts of large numbers of people who work on the river. To achieve the former you relate to 'other' with force and domination; Buber called such relationships 'I and It'. To achieve the latter you relate to others as equals – you listen, appreciate and develop mutually enhancing ways of behaving; Buber called such relationships 'I and Thou'. Both are needed, appropriate to the needs of the moment.

We oscillate between 'I–Thou' and 'I–It' thinking to integrate complex things

Martin Buber (1878–1965) was an Austrian-born Jewish philosopher best known for his philosophy of dialogue that identified two quite different ways of relating to people. He called them 'I and Thou', and 'I and It'. He argued that people mostly need 'I–It' relations, but quality of life in a community or society depends on the extent to which 'I–Thou' relations exist.

'I–Thou', and 'I–It' are *mindsets* – different expectations of how I relate to things around me.

'I–It', Buber maintains, sees things as unchanging products of the past – as objects. 'I–It' is an expectation that things other than me are concrete facts and I should relate to them in concrete, controlling ways, as you would to an emotionless machine. The 'I–It' mentality does not see others as complex, responsive, living organisms and does not entertain the thought of creatively interacting with them. 'I–It' distances myself from others and disallows interpretations other than mine.

'I–Thou' is quite different. This way of thinking sees others as interesting and responsive complex organisms. 'I–Thou' involves being alive in the present and engaging with others in ways that appreciate their beauty, complexity and potential. 'I–Thou' is a forward-looking encounter of one whole being with another from which new things can emerge.

The being does not have to be a *human* being, as Buber explains:

> I consider a tree. I can look on it as a picture: stiff column in a shock of light, or splash of green shot with the delicate blue and silver of the background. I can perceive it as movement: flowing veins on clinging, pressing pith, suck of the roots, breathing of the leaves, ceaseless commerce with earth and air . . . I can classify it in a species and study it as a type in its structure and mode of life. In all this the tree remains my object, occupies space and time . . . It can, however, also come about, if I have both will and grace, that in considering the tree I become bound up in relation to it. The tree is no longer It.

 Buber, M. (translated by Smith, R.G.). *I and Thou*. London: Bloomsbury Academic, 2013 (Kindle location 188–190)

We need both mindsets to develop trusted relationships – for 'I' to become 'we'.

We need both mindsets for transformation – to allow a new me to come into being.

We need both mindsets to integrate care and promote health – to develop shared stories across disciplinary and organisational boundaries.

To use both mindsets well we have to oscillate between them. 'I–Thou' helps me to play. 'I–It' helps me to control my environment.

The trouble is, people often use the two mindsets inappropriately, as witnessed by the child whose spoon misses their mouth because they are 'playing' with their food, and the parent who fails to play with the child because they are distracted by their own anxieties.

We oscillate between 'I–Thou' and 'I–It' thinking to live life forwards

In giving you receive
(Francis of Assisi)

St Francis' popular quote can be interpreted in a transactional way - if I give something the other will give me something back. This is an 'I-It' mindset. It can also be interpreted in a transformational way- the act of giving enriches me. Like giving a smile, I also smile inside. This is an 'I-Thou' mindset, not mechanistic but co-creative and healing.

Buber's 'I-Thou' interaction with a tree needed *'will and grace'* to *'become bound up in relation to'* it. An 'I-Thou' encounter requires me to dissolve into experiences; to lose sight of who I am. I re-emerge almost exactly the same person, but with new insights. I have moved my life story forwards – an incremental transformation. The people I share the experience with are similarly changed since we have intertwined parts of our identities. 'I' becomes 'we'.

Like the Buddhist concept of *mindfulness*, the Christian concept of *contemplation,* and religious festivals like Diwali and Caribbean carnivals, 'I-Thou' demands me to immerse in the experience rather than control it, and to play with others as equals. It requires me to give of myself, optimistically and trusting, without expecting anything specific in return. I receive things indirectly – trusted relationships, wisdom, love, stories, insight, a sense of belonging. The more I give, the more I receive.

The 'I-Thou' encounter is a spiritual experience. Mystics describe feeling 'bound up' in this way. But in more modest ways it happens every time I marvel at the beauty of a flower or a child, or laugh at the humour of a comedian, or feel the power of music, or smile at someone in the street. It happens every time I pause from my focused work to look around and appreciate the world beyond my immediate preoccupation.

One question is whether energy flows during 'I-Thou' encounters. Some say it does, like radio waves. Others say the effect is caused by hormones in our brains – Pert's 'Molecules of Emotion'. The answer may not matter. What matters is knowing that we can powerfully affect others, for good or bad, by the way we interact with them.

When I reach out to someone like Buber did with the tree and they *respond in kind*, that person is also open to an 'I-Thou' encounter. The person responds in a listening, co-creative way that enhances me – makes me feel alive, connected, loved, cared for, appreciated, noticed, useful, valuable, worthwhile, liked. . . . . Not an object.

But there is no guarantee that the other *will* respond in kind. If I approach someone with an 'I-Thou' mind-set and encounter an 'I-It' mind-set, it feels like extending a hand of friendship and receiving a slap in the face. It feels like being treated as an object.

Treating people as objects - as 'Its' - dehumanises them. This is what Marx called *'alienation', South Africa* called *'apartheid'* and generally is called un-caring, un-listening, thought-less. Yet it happens all the time. It is much easier to focus on self-interest and delusion than to see things in their fullness and work creatively with them. We can all fall into the trap of seeing only our own point of view and failing to put ourselves into the shoes of others.

We oscillate between 'I–Thou' and 'I–It' thinking to learn and change

The 'I–Thou' awareness state is not possible or desirable much of the time. Practical demands force a functional way of behaving. In addition, it is quite simply exhausting to always be so open. People need to purposefully move between 'I–It' and 'I–Thou' relations (and back again). This oscillation can be learned. Simple techniques like a deep breath, stretching, mantras and smiling can flick the switch.

Individuals can be broadly aware and narrowly focused at the same time. A GP can see diseases and life stories at the same time. An author deep in thought can instantly adjust to be fully there for someone who comes into the room, without losing their train of thought. A traveller can scan the street for opportunities and dangers without losing a step.

Oscillation between bigger pictures and focused tasks is also needed for organisations to learn and change. Lewin (Chapter 19) famously described 'freeze–unfreeze' as a requirement of a healthy organisation. This, now standard technique, involves periodically 'unfreezing' – standing back and reviewing past story, future vision and plans for the next stage; then again 'freezing' – everyone gets their heads down and does focused tasks until the next time to 'unfreeze'.

Oscillation between focused detail and broader systems is how people keep balanced in a complex moving world. It is how individuals learn and change. It is how organisations and systems learn and change.

It is how people avoid becoming stuck in a rut.

Kolb's learning cycle (Chapter 19) shows that individuals learn by oscillating between focused thinking and broad thinking in two dimensions – between concrete experience and abstract conceptualisation, and between active experimentation and reflective observation. He puts them together to describe a four-stage cycle of reflection and action. The same cycle of learning and change is used in audit, action research and organisational development. Kolb's learning cycle has multiple applications in community-oriented integrated care.

Similarly, Argyris and Schon (Chapter 19) describe a need to oscillate between three different kinds of learning – *single-loop learning* establishes facts; *double-loop learning* surfaces hidden truths; and *deutero-learning* finds new ways to continually learn and change ('learning how to learn'). A healthy organisation engages in ongoing cycles of learning and change that cover all three.

Any one aspect of learning on its own can lead in a poor direction. We find the best route by weighing up different kinds of evidence, debate between different perspectives and pilot testing. The best direction can be described as a 'leap of faith', 'vision', 'creativity' or 'gut instinct'. It is also a highly sophisticated process of weighing up different scenarios.

Both individuals and organisations move their lives forward through cycles of learning and change. Actions for change combines non-linear leaps of imagination and plodding, linear steps. Wisdom is finding the best combination; it comes through the language of learning.

Learning from and with others starts to appear as a useful answer to questions that at first sight may seem unrelated: 'What policy will stimulate, nourish and renew integrated care?' and the question 'How can I live a meaningful, healthy life?' The answer to each includes the same message – live life forwards with optimism, respect the past and take measured steps towards a healthy future vision, be always ready to learn and change and take occasional leaps of faith, appreciate the perspectives of others, remember your own story and develop it through networks of trusted relationships that help you to fit with the ever-changing world you encounter. Think 'I–Thou' as much as possible. *Be alive in the moment.*

Becoming locked in 'I–It' thinking prevents healthy forward movement

Many people are stuck in an 'I–It' way of thinking, at least in certain contexts. They lack the skill or the will to meaningfully engage with the world they encounter. Instead, they divert their energy to backward-looking control and combat, isolating themselves from the situation. They are projecting Berne's illusions; failing to master Erikson's states.

Here are furrowed brows on people with a 'broken record' of complaint playing inside their heads, people on mobile phones unable to see that the sun is shining, doctors with eyes glued to the computer screen unable to see that the patient is crying. In each of these situations, the actors lack the eyes to see the humanity of others. They fail to see everyday opportunities for fun and laughter, play, novelty, love and co-creation.

Fear and anxiety are common reasons for overdoing 'I–It' thinking. But not the only ones. Some do it as a learned habit that has never been successfully challenged. Some have arrested development through failure to pass a life stage. Some are unable to see beyond their need to protect their personal space, through illness, pain or being overwhelmed. Some have simply had too much success, and have never had reason to imagine themselves to be anything other than central to everything.

Many ideologies encourage 'I–It' thinking – individualism, consumerism, competition – all encourage functional efficiencies at the expense of human relationships. They all encourage the idea that everything is an established 'It' rather than a co-evolving 'Thou'.

Without 'I–Thou' to complement it, the 'I–It' mindset damages the person who holds it as much as those they interact with. They are unable to develop themselves because they live inside what Pope Francis described as 'soap bubbles' formed to retain a 'culture of comfort, which makes us think only of ourselves, makes us insensitive to the cries of other people . . . [resulting in] globalized indifference'.

  Ivereigh, A. *The Great Reformer: Francis and the making of a radical pope.* Crow's Nest, NSW: Allen & Unwin, 2014 (Kindle location 155–163)

The trouble is, entrenched 'I–It' thinking is difficult to break out of. It requires humility to acknowledge my mistakes and change my opinions. Such changes can challenge my sense of self, causing an existential crisis. Merely listening to different perspectives can be exhausting. It is much easier to remain locked in my own way of thinking, and from there try to control and blame others, than to engage positively with a range of people I little understand or care about. It is much easier to construct short-term stand-alone projects and falsely believe that they will transform a whole system, than to chart a course for genuine whole system transformation.

Crises can cause people to break out of chronic 'I–It' thinking. Many only wake up to the need to appreciate others and work creatively with them when things have got really bad – a serious illness, an ecological disaster, manifest injustice. An earthquake led to the Pegasus project (collaborative primary care) in New Zealand. Injustice in South America led to *liberation theology* and Freire's *critical consciousness*.

Relying on crises is not a good strategy. Instead, it is better to be familiar with a science of complex co-adaptation. This explains why uncertainty and courage and adventure and hope and humour and play and mistakes and forgiveness and care are all part of a healthy life.

One thing we learn is that words themselves are not enough to describe what is happening.

Words are co-constructed to give voice to experience

Buber makes great emphasis on appreciative silence in 'I–Thou' relations.

One reason for silence is the need to listen more than speak when trying to understand others. Another reason is that words are not adequate for movements into the future. Words are another form of 'It' – they were made in the past and may not describe the future.

Taylor agrees with Habermas that we construct our sense of self through exchange in *language*. Through discussion we negotiate words that describe our shared experience and this informs our identities and culture. It doesn't happen in the linear way described here. Instead, experience, words, identity, culture all develop at the same time in swirls of interaction and sense-making that only with hindsight is understandable in words. In the present moment, it just feels meaningful. Words are yet to come. Stories are yet to be told.

 Taylor, C. *Sources of the Self: the making of the modern identity*. Cambridge: Cambridge University Press, 1989 (p. 509)

Shotter describes it well. He wrote:

> most of the time we do not fully understand what another person says. Indeed in practice, shared understandings occur only occasionally, if they occur at all. And when they do, it is by people testing and checking each others' talk, by them questioning and challenging it, reformulating and elaborating it, and so on . . . Primarily, it seems, they are responding to each other's utterances in an attempt to link their practical activities in with those of the others around them; and in these attempts at co-ordinating their activities, people are constructing one or another kind of social relationship.

> (p. 1)

 Shotter, J. *Conversational Realities: constructing life through language*. London: Sage, 1993

Words describe the past (and not often reliably). They shape but do not define the future.

Bird-nesting belief systems explain the need for incremental transformations

People accumulate a lot of words. Born from personal experience, theories, assumptions, imagination, and especially from those we trust, we accumulate a personal collection of words, theories, beliefs and ideas that we use to make sense of the world.

Leavey calls this 'bird-nesting belief system'. I pick words, ideas, theories from here and there to make the 'nest' I live in – my 'home', my 'comfort zone', my identity. The 'twigs' in my nest give me mental models to interpret the world I encounter; taking twigs away challenges my sense of self. They give me eyes to see some things and be blind to others. They make me behave the way I do. They guide my every action, irrespective of whether they achieve what I want. Often the same person has conflicting mental models; for example the adolescent trait of refusing to listen to others, yet also expecting to be told what to do.

 Leavey, C. *Why Do Women Not Attend for Cervical Smear Appointments? A participatory action research approach in liverpool general practice* (PhD dissertation). Liverpool: John Moores University: 2000, pp. 252–253

The link between my nest of beliefs and my sense of self explains why transformational change is so painful. I have to replace parts of my 'nest' – parts of me – to learn and change. It explains why the things I 'see' have more to do with what my nest allows me to see than with what there is to be seen. It explains *cognitive dissonance* – favouring my cherished beliefs over the truth. It explains *projection* – attributing traits to someone else that are more truthfully my own. It explains *prejudice* – pre-judging situations, before I really know.

Of course nests change all the time. Like decorating a house, when done bit by bit you hardly notice that it is becoming quite different from what it once was. This is why sequential cycles of inter-organisational learning and change is a better strategy to transform a whole system than periodic 'big bang' revolutions. Although both have their place.

One reason why integration doesn't happen enough is that different individuals, disciplines and institutions live in different places and lack opportunities to transform their 'nests' in synchrony. Practitioners lead research *or* they lead development. Institutions lead organisational development *or* service improvements. Different philosophical traditions lead physical, social, mental *or* spiritual health initiatives. They all lead, but they don't link.

It is understandable why they don't link. Each body of knowledge is vast; to avoid being overwhelmed we create boundaries. Boundaries obstruct links. Boundaries include carving up the work into separate disciplines and even being trained in different locations – different disciplines do not even bump into each other. These boundaries, coupled with an over-abundance of 'I–It' thinking makes it amazing that so much works as well as it does.

The way to overcome the divisive nature of boundaries has been known throughout history – you have to cross them. From the ancient Tower of Babel to contemporary marriage guidance counsellors the same lesson has to be learned and re-learned – we need to listen to those who are different from us and appreciate what they have to offer. We need shared adventures in which we develop shared stories. This is not possible if we lack the opportunity, or the will, or the skill, or the confidence to reach out a hand of friendship.

This signals a core skill of team players within integrated care – to facilitate *intergenerational learning* – to learn from and with those who are different from us, and act on that learning. We need to be prepared to 'travel a mile in the shoes' of others and have the humility to learn from the experience and see the things we need to change in ourselves. Then we need the determination to make those changes, and repeat the process again and again, becoming wise through cycles of learning and change. Being able to learn and change in synchrony with others is a skill that everyone needs – health-care leaders and practitioners, patients and indeed every citizen, at every age.

To make this happen at scale:

* Individuals need to be reflective practitioners, able to relate their daily experiences to the bigger journeys that are undertaking.
* Organisations need to be learning organisations, able to facilitate cycles of inter-disciplinary collaborative reflection and coordinated action.
* Whole systems need feedback loops and connected learning spaces that enliven all parts of the 'body'.
* Policy needs to apply principles of learning in everything: inter-disciplinary team-learning, organisational learning, learning communities, learning systems.

Part V continues the exploration of theories that help to understand how to build trusted relationships and healthy communities – network theory (Chapter 17), transactional analysis (Chapter 18), learning organisations (Chapter 19), whole society participation (Chapter 20).

Narrative unity shows how to promote health in complex situations

The health of an individual depends on their relationships

No one stands alone. People define themselves by their networks of relationships. Primary care must help people to develop strong relationships within families and communities.

Relationships need mutual appreciation, energising shared projects and touch

When relationships become functional arrangements, the spark goes out of them. The sense of 'we' fragments into separate 'I's. Relationships grow through new adventures. They need physical contact, whether the intimacy of lovers, the hug of a friend or a formal handshake.

People need to continually re-write their life stories for them to remain positive and coherent

When people review their life stories they might see past experiences that make their sense of self seem fragmented or vulnerable; rewriting the interpretation of those experiences can help them to become more healthy.

Everyone needs to be a team player

Team players see the value of different perspectives and adapt their personal behaviours to fit well with those of others. Team players help people to listen to each other, value different perspectives and constantly reappraise their own views.

Reminiscence helps people to feel alive

Getting an elderly person to review their life story helps them to again feel young – perhaps watching old films, reviewing old photographs or listening to music they once danced to.

Music, metaphor and dance are more in tune with the world than words

Words pick out certain aspects from a world that is more complex than words can fully appreciate. Music, metaphor and dance are better at appreciating the dynamic and complex nature of the world because they reveal different ways to harmonise different contributions.

Life transitions are moments when stories can transform

The first day of school, adolescence, entering the world of work, a first baby, illness, retirement. These are moments when people are forced to come out of their shells, so they *may* be more open to transformational change – before the shutters come down again.

In life transitions get your affairs in order

It is important to mark major life transitions, and at those times finish past business - reconcile old hurts; say goodbye to those you are leaving behind; get your affairs in order.

Anxiety is a natural reaction to a threat to coherence

People feel anxious when they feel out of control. Internal anxiety causes external aggression. By gently facing the causes of their anxiety, people can reduce the harm they cause to themselves and to others, and emerge stronger and wiser.

Everyday actions can be healing

Merely listening to someone – really listening – makes someone feel valued as a whole person within a community. Things like remembering things that matter to someone can enhance their sense of health. Confronting life stresses positively can improve health.

Relevance of narrative unity to community-oriented integrated care

Narrative unity signals a world of bewildering complexity where everything is constantly adapting to everything else in ways that words alone cannot explain. Nobody knows what they don't know, yet many believe that they have nothing else to learn. Few fully listen to others, nor even to themselves, and instead their actions are often guided by reliving past difficulties instead of engaging with their present reality. Everyone picks out facts and fantasies that fit with the stories they want to tell, project onto others attributes that are more truthfully their ow, and avoid conversations with people who do not share their views. This creates multiple incompatible 'truths' and 'silo-operating' that obstruct harmonious working.

And when someone wakes up to these everyday maladies, they discover that the more they know, the more they know they don't know, causing a different sense of impotence.

If integration is to work, there need to be routine processes to gently challenge behaviours. We need cross-boundary learning and change to be routine daily activities throughout whole systems of care. These need to allow different story-strands to be valued and become entwined, building relationships and communities in multiple directions. Families, schools, universities, workplaces, faith groups, voluntary groups and all other aspects of society needs to promote this in their own domains of influence, and support the work of others.

Navigating it well requires us to *travel hopefully* mindful that anything can happen. Individual and collective learning need to be a way of life, as reflective practitioners in learning organisations and learning communities.

Here are skills a healthy person needs to continually develop. He/she is able to:

- *be alive in the moment* – dis-eases can challenge that sense of vitality, yet they can also be used creatively to enhance it
- *adventure in an uncertain world*, able to live life forwards with optimism, see whole stories as well as individual facts, inquire into complex situations, learn from experience and use all of these to turn bad into good
- *be a team player*, able to dip in and out of different kinds of project, making timely and synchronous contributions that make wholes more than the sum of the parts
- *be a life-long, life-wide learner*, able to reflect, challenge myself and others to change our behaviours and ways of thinking, and to learn from and with those who have different life experiences
- *be resilient*, able to bend like a reed in the wind without breaking under pressure and remain centred when things are turbulent – surfing the waves of life

This dynamic image of reality is poorly understood by laboratory 'quantitative' approaches to inquiry. More trustworthy approaches are discussed in Chapter 16.

Chapter 16

Three paradigms of inquiry illuminate evolving stories

Key message: Different approaches to inquiry reveal different things.

In this chapter:

- Medical science promotes fragmentation
- Linear and complexity lenses are wrongly separated
- Research is illumination
- Challenges to positivism
- Simple rules?
- Guba's three paradigms of knowledge
- Crystallisation of meaning versus triangulation of evidence
- Why are Guba's three paradigms so pervasive?
- Relevance of Guba's three paradigms to community-oriented integrated care

Medical science promotes fragmentation

> Most songs are about love but it just won't plot on a bar graph.
>
> (Author original quote)

The emergence of 'Newtonian' science in the seventeenth century permitted unprecedented control of the world. It imagines the world to be made up of separate particles that can be examined in isolation from each other and interact with other particles in direct linear ways. It led to the agricultural and industrial revolutions from 1750 onwards that made Britain 'great'. Scientific method quickly became adopted in all aspects of life to assess situations and justify actions, for example through research methods like the *randomised controlled trial*.

In Western societies, the authority of science increasingly replaced the authority of the church to guide actions. Insidiously, the notion that life is made up of individual lumps of truth replaced the notion that life is a mystery within which different truths are connected by divine purpose. This concrete image of reality is the 'scientific paradigm' termed *positivism*.

One example of the belief that life is naturally separated into different compartments is 'Cartesian dualism' – body and mind are separate, concrete entities. René Descartes (1596–1650), often called the father of modern philosophy, and Isaac Newton (1643–1727), often called the father of modern science, were contemporaries. Their insights led to a mechanistic image of the world. Their ideas showed engineers how to build aeroplanes and doctors how to treat diseases. Modern evidence-based medicine is built on their theories.

One problem with the Newton/Descartes mental model is that it stimulates fragmentation. It focuses on the direct 'effects' of 'causes' without seeing the inter-dependence of particles and their co-adaptation to each other. Through Newton's lens things don't change except in superficial ways. People exist as isolated commodities. Relationships do not exist except as mechanical functions. It encourages hierarchical and controlling models, and causes conflict and prejudice. Love, team-working and integration are invisible to this way of thinking.

This does not mean that linear theories and models are wrong. It merely means that they are limited to isolated linear phenomena – the immediate effects of single actions. They pick out from the complexity of the world those aspects that are amenable to objective validation. Other theories and models are needed to reveal the web of relationships that make an individual who they are. Other theories are needed to reveal the interactions between different people that co-create a trusted relationship. Other theories are needed for community-oriented integrated care.

Linear and complexity lenses are wrongly separated

The belief that the world is naturally made up of distinct particles that impact on each other in linear and hierarchical ways goes back much further than Newton and Descartes. Both Plato and Aristotle believed in a natural hierarchy of order. The biblical assertion that humans have dominion over the world is a hierarchical notion. Indeed, the very belief that individuals have a personal sense of self is a compartmentalised idea.

Descartes, Newton, Smith, Plato and Aristotle did not solely believe in linear interactions between separate particles. They all had profound spiritual beliefs. They compartmentalised their dual beliefs, or had them compartmentalised for them by others – mystery and complexity aspects are managed by God or Nature; linear and controlling aspects are managed by man.

Other great historical thinkers had ideas that were more complex than popularly believed. By 'survival of the fittest', Charles Darwin meant survival of the most adaptable, rather than the most ruthless, as his example of the giraffe illustrates. By 'the market', Adam Smith did not envisage remote electronic transactions, but inter-human haggling that has unpredictable outcomes, as though 'led by an invisible hand to promote an end which was no part of his intention'.

 Smith, A. *An Inquiry into the Nature and Causes of the Wealth of Nations.* London: Alex Murray & Son; Book 4, Chap II (p. 354), 1871

More: Donabedian presents structure, process and outcome as a linear progression when his own examples show that they are mutually inter-dependent. Maslov presents his *hierarchy of needs* with self-actualisation at the top and functional things like food and shelter lower down – yet in reality, self-actualisation is present in all types of human experience, including when most basic needs are unmet, as is witnessed in the self-organisation and creativity within shanty towns.

Linear and complexity thinking are always there. It is the mistaken belief that linear thinking is more important that airbrushes out complexity. In truth, neither is more or less important than the other. They are different things, like air and water are different things; more of one does not overcome the need for the others. Linear thinking and complexity thinking are the yin and yang of Western thought. When used in complementary ways they breathe life into each other – one deals with the 'hard' things that can be seen and measured and controlled; the other with the 'soft' things that help people to creatively interact and co-evolve. One deals with the concrete and immediate; the other with the abstract and visionary. All relationships, including integrated care, need both, intertwined, like a tune needs a beat.

Lack of understanding that the 'hard' and the 'soft' need to be intertwined may explain why society often designs structures that keep them apart, without mechanisms to integrate them. Research and development, public health and primary care, doctors and nurses, policy and education, academics and practitioners, specialists and generalists – they are all kept in separate boxes. They live in different institutions, appeal to different libraries of knowledge, use different languages and often fail to communicate except in the most perfunctory ways. Yet they need each other to be effective.

Compartmentalisation and control look neat but they don't make things work well. The challenge for everyone is to maintain systems that truly make things work. This means systems that enable ongoing, syncretic interweaving of ideas and co-adaptation across disciplines. That is, cycles of collaborative learning and coordinated change.

Research is illumination

> What we observe is not nature itself, but nature exposed to our method of questioning
>
> (Werner Heisenberg)

Heisenberg reminds us that different lenses reveal different aspects of the world. The success of the (positivist) scientific paradigm in the last 400 years has led to the idea that it is always the best lens. For example, the randomised controlled trial is often considered to be the 'gold standard' of research irrespective of what you are researching.

The term *paradigm* was made popular by Thomas Kuhn in the 1960s as a way to describe shifts of understanding that bring new ways of thinking about reality. The origin of the term has a more general meaning. It comes from a Greek word meaning 'pattern' or 'model' or 'set of ideas' or 'something to point at'. It has been used in a subjective sense – the 'paradigm of a perfect woman' (useful for marketing), an objective sense – 'the world is round' (useful for air travel) and a practical sense – 'the world is flat' (useful for road travel).

Paradigms should not be set one above the other in a hierarchy of truth. They are *lenses*, *metaphors* or *mental models* that see things that resonate with that way of looking, in the same way that a green lens sees green things and filters out red.

As Parlett and Hamilton point out, *research is illumination*. Different paradigms shine different lights on reality. What you see depends on the light you shine.

 Parlett, M. and Hamilton, E. Evaluation as illumination: a new approach to the study of innovatory programs. Occasional paper. Edinburgh University, Centre for Research in the Educational Sciences. Nuffield Foundation: London, 1972

The question should not be 'what paradigm of inquiry is the best?', but 'what combination of paradigms is most useful to illuminate the things we want to understand?'

A paradigm of inquiry is an approach to asking questions, a school of inquiry that has rules about rigour and validity. In recent years there have been two broad main inquiry paradigms – *quantitative* and *qualitative*. Things you can count and things you can't.

So what is wrong with believing that you can precisely count everything?

Challenges to positivism

Until recently, positivist science, with its emphasis on machine-like precision and linear interactions between measurable particles, was considered by many to be the only believable lens to look at the world. As Skinner pointed out, this has dramatically changed:

> Times have certainly changed . . . The empiricist and positivist citadels of English-speaking social philosophy have been threatened and undermined by successive waves of hermeneutics, structuralists, post-empiricists, deconstructionists and other invaded hoards . . . Perhaps the most significant transformation has been the widespread reaction against the assumption that the natural sciences offer an adequate or even a relevant model for the practice of the social disciplines . . . and the positivist contention that all successful explanations must conform to the same deductive model must be fundamentally misconceived.

 Skinner, Q. (ed.) *The Return of Grand Theory in the Human Sciences.* Cambridge: Cambridge University Press, 1985 (p. 6)

Challenge to the idea that everything of value can be counted has long come from the social sciences. More recently, challenges have come from the natural sciences, including biology, physics, neuroscience and mathematics. For example, Candace Pert has demonstrated that microscopic polypeptides link the body and the mind, providing a mechanism for something as simple as a smile to affect the physical functioning or someone else. She shows that the human body behaves as Darwin predicted – integration is not achieved by the brain in a hierarchy of direct control, but through vast numbers of multiple-way interactions and feedback loops that allow all cells in a body to co-evolve in synchronous ways. The human body behaves like a *learning organisation*.

 Pert, C. *Molecules of Emotion.* London: Simon & Schuster (Pocket Books), 1999

Complexity theory shows that multiple interactions lead to self-organisation through co-adaptation. It reveals predictable patterns, termed 'fractals', within complex situations that are real only to those involved. For example, the swirl of water around a plughole and the square route of a negative number both reveal predictable patterns that defy simple laws of cause and effect; and the predictability disappears when you interfere from the outside – including when you try to measure them.

Voices from within general practice have argued the urgent need for a science that better understands things that are complex and canot be simply counted:

> the current explanatory model in medicine, based ultimately on scientific positivism, is no longer sufficient on its own to equip the professionals working in the field.
>
> (p. xi)

 Sweeney, K. and Griffiths, F. (eds) *Complexity and Healthcare: An Introduction.* Abingdon: Radcliffe Medical Press, 2002

> complexity theory draws from the fundamental organising principles of nature . . . It sees the world as a system . . . that is non-linear . . . and dynamic . . . Organisations are viewed as structures that not only bring people together to discharge specific functions but also places where people make sense of their lives.
>
> (p. xv)

 Kernick, D. (ed.) *Complexity and Healthcare Organization*: A View from the Street. Abingdon: Radcliffe Medical Press, 2004

Stacey and Plesk have popularised the term *complex adaptive system* that is now used worldwide to inform health-care strategy.

Introducing a series of books on the topic, Stacey writes:

> The aim of this series is to give expression to a particular way of speaking about complexity in organizations, one that emphasises self-referential, reflexive nature of humans, the essentially responsive and participative nature of human processes of relating and the radical unpredictability of their evolution. It draws on the complexity sciences, which can be brought together in many ways to form a whole spectrum of theories of human organization.
>
> (p. ix)

 Stacey, R., Griffin, D. and Shaw, P. *Complexity and Management: Fad or radical challenge to systems thinking?* London: Routledge, 2000

Plesk explains, when commenting on health-care developments in the USA:

> It is more helpful to think like a farmer than an engineer or an architect in designing a health care system . . . the farmer simply creates the conditions under which a good crop is possible . . . relatively simple rules can lead to complex, emergent, innovative system behaviour . . . Simple rules for human complex adaptive systems tend to be of three types: 1) General Pointing, 2) Prohibitions, 3) Resource or permission providing . . . Rather than agonizing over plans, the goal is to generate a 'good enough plan' and begin to observe what happens. Then, modifications can occur in an evolutionary fashion.

 Plesk, P. Redesigning health care with insights from the science of complex adaptive systems. In *Crossing the Quality Chasm*. Washington, DC: National Academy Press, 2001, pp. 314–317

Plesk suggests that even if complex and emerging things can't be counted, people can engage with them by obeying 'simple rules'.

Simple rules?

The notion of 'simple rules' to understand complex behaviour between living things found prominence in the 1987 paper by Craig Reynolds in which he electronically simulated the flocking behaviour of birds (termed 'Boids'). The appearance of birds flocking in nature can be simulated by programming electronic boids to obey three rules:

1 Steer to avoid crowding local flockmates
2 Steer towards the average heading of local flockmates
3 Steer to move toward the average position (center of mass) of local flockmates

 Boids. https://en.wikipedia.org/wiki/Boids

Whether these rules reflect what is going on in the mind of a bird is less interesting than the idea than we can guide people to engage with uncertain and complex situation by requiring them to follow some simple, concrete and measurable 'rules', without them having to know anything at all about complexity theory. This is useful for policy for integrated working.

We use simple rules all the time to engage with complex things. For example:

• Drive on the agreed side of the road (left or right; it doesn't matter which)
• Do unto others as you would have them do unto you
• Think positive
• Do your best

Some simple rules for policy for integrated working are described in a box at the beginning of Part I – 'Policy that supports community-oriented integrated care'.

One simple rule that might help people to see dynamic things in complex situations is: *Use quantitative and qualitative inquiry at the same time.*

One difficulty with this is that qualitative inquiry is usually defined as anything that isn't quantitative. But you can't define something in terms of what it isn't. This begs the question: "What is qualitative inquiry?"

Guba's three paradigms of knowledge

The speed with which understanding of qualitative research is developing can be witnessed by comparing the 1994 and 2000 editions of the *Handbook of Qualitative Research*. They reveal a shift in considering qualitative research to be anything that isn't quantitative to approaches to inquiry that make different assumptions about the nature of the world, and the relationship of researchers to it (termed *ontology* and *epistemology*).

 Denzin, N.K. and Lincoln, Y.S. (eds) *Handbook of Qualitative Research*. Thousand Oaks, CA: Sage, 1994

Denzin, N.K. and Lincoln, Y.S. (eds) *Handbook of Qualitative Research* Second Edition. Thousand Oaks, CA: Sage, 2000

In 1982, Egon Guba convened a conference in San Francisco to analyse three paradigms of inquiry that had emerged out of naïve positivism – *post-positivism*, *critical theory* and *constructivism*. In the *Paradigm Dialog*, 32 authors contributed to the book that Guba edited to describe these paradigms.

The box below describes the ontological and epistemological assumptions made by these three paradigms. Post-positivism examines individual countable facts, for example the effect of a self-help website on avoiding hospital admissions. Critical theory looks at the hidden connections that exist between different factors, for example social networks that help people to stay out of hospital. Constructivism looks at emergence from dynamic interaction; for example deciding a set of actions to avoid hospital admission after a family conference.

 Guba, E.G. (ed.) *The Paradigm Dialog*. Newbury Park, CA: Sage, 1990

These three inquiry paradigms, together, describe what it means to 'use quantitative and qualitative inquiry at the same time'. Chapter 11 describes inquiry methods that relate to each of these three paradigms. They can be applied in research, evaluation and audit.

Ontological and epistemological assumptions made by different paradigms

(Extract from partner book – *Integrating Primary Health Care: Leading, managing, facilitating*)

Post-positivism expects the world to be ordered simply and to be predictable. Entities really exist, unchanging and irrespective of other things. This ontological assumption is 'critical realist'. Truth is like a nugget of gold waiting to be recognised. I know it is there because tests detect its objective presence (its epistemology is dualist-objectivist). Its methodology is experimental-manipulative – a question or hypothesis is stated in advance in propositional form and subjected to empirical tests under controlled conditions. This approach uses research methods, such as experiments, in which features of interest are named in advance, measured, and counted. Validity requires a statistical difference between these numbers. This theory has no power to reveal context (discrete features are counted in isolation from other things), and no power to reveal novelty (things must be named in advance). The French philosopher Auguste Comte coined the term positivism in the 19th century. It was a reaction against the theological and metaphysical understandings of knowledge that predated it. The new science was empowering, allowing people to predict what would happen in simple situations. For example, travellers can trust the structural integrity of airplanes, and doctors can know what treatments are better at curing diseases.

Critical (Social) Theory, or 'ideologically oriented inquiry', reveals the context of a phenomenon. As with positivism its ontology is critical realist – truth is still expected to be there, but hidden by more superficial or transient truths. The researcher considers different perspectives and meanings that are not immediately obvious. Its epistemology is subjectivist in that critical theory values what people know from experience. Its methodology is dialogic – people of different perspectives debate the rights and wrongs of different versions of the truth to remove 'false consciousness' and arrive at a better version of the truth. This approach uses research methods, such as case studies, that focus on a phenomenon within its real-life context. Validity requires concordance between different perceptions (termed triangulation) that pinpoints the so-called real truth. The origins of critical theory are attributed to the German philosopher Jürgen Habermas, who maintained that our understandings of the world are distorted because we are blind to much of what is relevant.

Constructivism reveals novelty and innovation and is associated with John Shotter's concept of *social constructionism*. Constructivism maintains that truth is co-created from interaction between the inquirer and the inquired . . . who 'become fused into a single (monist) entity'. For example, gravity is a manifestation of the attractive properties of matter; love is a manifestation of shared meaning between people. These interactions have not a realist, but a relativist ontology – true-to-those-involved. The ontological-epistemological distinction is obliterated in constructivism, because what is really there and the relation of the observer-participant to it are different versions of the same question. This approach uses research methods such as appreciative inquiry and participatory action research which facilitate mutual learning, emergent understandings, and consensus. Validity requires consensus from different perspectives (termed crystallisation of meaning).

Crystallisation of meaning versus triangulation of evidence

The test to establish if something is true from a positivist or critical theory perspective is 'triangulation'. It's an objective test. To establish the height of a mountain you look at it from three different angles to triangulate where it 'really' is *objectively*. This is very useful when you are looking for one specific object.

But asking if a garden is beautiful is subjective. There is no one objective truth to triangulate. Beauty is 'in the eye of the beholder' – one person will find flowers beautiful, another trees, another water features, and different people will consider different layouts and combinations to be more or less beautiful. And each person will change their views over time.

To establish what a group or community considers to be beautiful you have to ask the people to reflect on what they think. They may not have a view at first. Then you get them to critique their views, through discussion with others and testing them out. This results in an emerging truth, termed *crystallisation of meaning* – like a solid crystal that emerges from a saturated solution, truth emerges from the dialectic.

Janesick, V.J. The choreography of qualitative research design: minuets, improvisations, and crystallization. Chapter 13 in *Handbook of Qualitative Research*. Second edition. Thousand Oaks, CA: Sage, 2000, pp. 391–392

You can triangulate whether the prevalence of a disease has reduced, but you can't triangulate whether a community is healthy. This requires crystallisation of meaning. Just as an individual brings their life story into view through personal reflection and checking their facts with others, a community forms a consensus about its community spirit by a similar process of group reflection and testing things out.

You can easily experience crystallisation of meaning – walk in a garden and reflect on what you smell and see and feel. Ask yourself what these experiences mean to you as a whole.

Why are Guba's three paradigms so pervasive?

Guba's three paradigms are lurking everywhere. They are not just about inquiry or evaluation. Different theories and languages reinvent a very similar trio of concepts. Moreover, they are usually found to be complementary and inter-dependent, rather than alternatives or contradictory:

- *Post-positivism* reveals individual factors.
- *Critical theory* reveals links between factors.
- *Constructivism* reveals co-adaptation and transformation.

Positivism bears comparison with 'top-down' development – direct and certain.

Critical theory bears comparison with 'bottom-up' development – bringing together an array of interconnected pieces.

Constructivism bears comparison with 'whole-system' development – complex co-adaptations.

The paradigms can be found in Berne's ego states for human interaction – 'parent' (authoritative), 'adult' (considers different views), 'child' (playful). They can be found in three types of organisational learning – 'single-loop', 'double-loop' and 'deutero-learning'; and three types of complexity – 'simple', 'complicated' and 'complex'; and three teaching styles – 'didactic', 'Socratic' and 'experiential'.

They can even be found in Jesus' three faces of the divine – 'Father', 'Son' and 'Spirit'.

Four hundred years before Jesus, Plato described a similar trio – *reason, appetite* and *spirit* – as three natures of the soul. Three different *desires* vying with one another.

 Plato. *The Republic*. 435–444 (208–222). Chatham: Guild Publishing. 1990

The observation that these three ways of thinking crop up in different traditions suggests that they might be fundamental properties of the world, or of words, or of our minds. If this is true, they must be important to all endeavours that wish to integrate parts and wholes.

It is intriguing to speculate why these paradigms are so universal. Maybe Plato and Jesus have profoundly affected the construction of ideas in the Western world? Or maybe they are intrinsic to the nature of the world or humanity or thought or words or something else essential?

I favour the explanation that whenever someone feels himself or herself to be alive he or she is aware of three simultaneous truths:

1   I know that I am a separate unique individual.
2   I know that I am a set of different parts that need to connect to make a whole.
3   The energy that binds these parts and wholes together makes it all work.

If these three truths are apparent to me every time I am aware of being alive, no wonder they are deeply embedded in the way we think. No wonder people rediscover them when they think deeply about anything. If this is the explanation, they may also be recognisable by those who speak languages that were not influenced by ancient Greek, Aramaic and Latin.

Whatever the explanation, the degree to which Guba's paradigms are recognisable by different traditions presents an opportunity to integrate very different efforts for health. Different kinds of people – scientists, artists, spiritualists, medical and non-medical practitioners, people of faith, atheists and agnostics – are likely to share an ambition for healthy individuals, healthy communities and systems that make them relevant to each other. In their different languages each will recognise the simultaneous value of facts, hidden connections and emergence.

Relevance of Guba's three paradigms to community-oriented integrated care

Guba reminds us that every situation has *simple*, *complicated* and *complex* aspects that are illuminated by different ways of looking at the world. Integrated care needs to use all three ways of looking, most of the time, to build healthy individuals and healthy communities.

If Guba's three paradigms in combination *always* illuminate different and useful aspects of the world, the implications are breath-taking. For example:

• Political stances should be less described as left and right 'wings', and more different kind of balance between top-down, bottom-up and participatory approaches to policy.
• All three lenses should be used to research, evaluate and audit.
• Doctors should use them to understand illness and health, individuals and organisations.
• School children should learn them as core skills to adventure skilfully in a complex world and appreciate things beyond their personal interest and imagination.

These three paradigms shine different kinds of light on the past and the future and the present moment. Their insights are integrated through stories rather than hierarchies of importance. They explain why there is a non-linear link between research and development, and between learning and change. We need them in combination to see beyond the superficial – things that move and things that are inter-relational. We need them to evaluate anything complex – learning organisations, community development, parenting, end-of-life care, and so on.

Part V describes theories – networks, transactional analysis, and learning organisations – that use these three paradigms of inquiry to develop community-oriented integrated care.

Exercise

Stand in an outside place – a street, a park, etc. Look all around, turning full circle, to see all the different objects you recognise. Have a guess of how many objects you can see – 5? 50? 500? 5,000? Walk a few steps and observe how everything changes in relationship to everything else. What new things can you see, and feel? You are observing the simplest example of adaptation – everything changes because you have moved.

Now, look at people. See how each person moves in ways that make sense to him or her. Observe the ways they adapt to each other as they walk along – moving aside (or not), smiling or scowling, initiating conversations, and so on. You are observing complex co-adaptation.

Part V

Community-oriented integrated care – making it work

In Part V:

Who might find Part V useful?
The image to support Part V: Illuminating stories with complementary lenses
Introduction to Part V: incremental transformations
Box: Vision, metaphors, theories, principles, methods
Chapter 17: Networks for complicated journeys. *Network Theory* shows how to design a system that people can easily navigate and also have creative adventures within. A railway network needs: a) Nodes (stations and junctions) where different routes connect, b) Timetables and maps, and c) Trains that arrive on time. These are *mechanical aspects* of a network. They also need waiting rooms, restaurants and other places where passengers can interact with others, learn from them and review their travel plans. These are *living system* aspects. Integrated care needs both.
Chapter 18: Developing team players and systems-thinkers. *Transactional analysis* shows how to interact creatively with others to develop trusted relationships. It highlights three 'ego states' – 'parent', 'adult' and 'child'. When performing a functional task, like treating a disease, a one-dimension Adult-Adult or Parent-Child transaction is all that is needed. Human conversations that build trusted relationships require more sophisticated interactions, called 'games'. A 'good game' concludes a positive punch-line of 'I'm OK; You're OK' – conclusions have been negotiated; each demonstrates appreciation of the other; they have moved on their shared story. 'Bad games' diminish both/all players.
Chapter 19: Learning organisations build teams and communities. *Organisational learning* theory shows how organisations as well as individuals can learn and change to transform whole systems. It shows how to develop vibrant communities. Learning organisations facilitate cycles of inter-organisational learning and change that include stakeholder events and collaborative improvement projects.
Chapter 20: Public health and primary care – an essential partnership. This chapter describes how public health and general practice should work together to engage all citizens of their responsibilities to contribute to integrated care and health promotion. All sectors of society need to align their work for health and care to the boundaries of local health communities, to enhance each other's effects.

Who might find Part V useful?

This part is written for those who want to know how to build *equal relationships* and *high performing teams*, including those who design and lead integrated care and integrated health promotion, and those who want to improve their own relationships.

The part responds to the challenges of Part IV that describe the enormous complexity of the world as everyone adapts to everyone else. Health and integrated working are not passive things. You have to make an effort. You have to reach out to others, learn from them and negotiate with them. You have to continually transform yourself to remain true to yourself. If you stay stuck in your past, you shrivel.

The part revisits Guba's three paradigms (Chapter 16) that bring into view three quite different ways of thinking about reality. Each is useful for different aspects of change. *Linear change* copies an established pattern of behaviour; e.g. a model of health promotion. *Emergent change* makes new links between existing things; e.g. a new way to communicate between existing teams. *Transformational change* alters the nature of relationships and stories; e.g. team-working rather than individual working.

The image to support Part V: Illuminating stories with complementary lenses

This image combines the idea of *narrative unity* (Chapter 15 – everyone seeks to make their life stories coherent) with Guba's paradigms of inquiry (Chapter 16 – three different assumptions about reality). Individuals develop meaningful life stories by considering three different kinds of information in the light of their past history and their hopes for the future.

On the left is the story so far – of an individual or a group. On the right is their future vision. Connecting the past and the future is a 'life script' – how the story-holders expect the story to unfold. The life script is what makes us notice some things and be blind to others.

The three 'lights' in the middle are Guba's three paradigms of inquiry. These see different aspects of the emerging story. *Positivism* sees separate, countable 'facts' – e.g. hospital admissions, care plans and death rates. *Critical theory* reveals the strands that connect different facts – e.g. relationships, anxiety and ambitions. *Constructivism* sees new things being co-constructed – e.g. Development trust or fear from life experiences.

By discussing what the different lenses reveal about an experience, an individual or group can bring into view a range of insights about possible actions. They 'play' with these ideas – bouncing them off each other so each stimulates compatible changes in the others, to both fit well together and to co-create new directions. From this they conclude a shared plan – steps they think are likely to move in the direction of the overall vision.

Then, of course, they need the skill, opportunity and will to take the next steps.

The image reminds us that the future cannot be simply dictated by the past. Research ('R') and development ('D') are *not* related in simple, 'linear' ways. Good policy comes from systematically generating different kinds of evidence and making sense of them as a whole, through discussion and testing things out.

The image reminds us that reality is not a static thing. What we see is a fleeting glimpse of more complex stories-in-evolution. When things look still we are merely

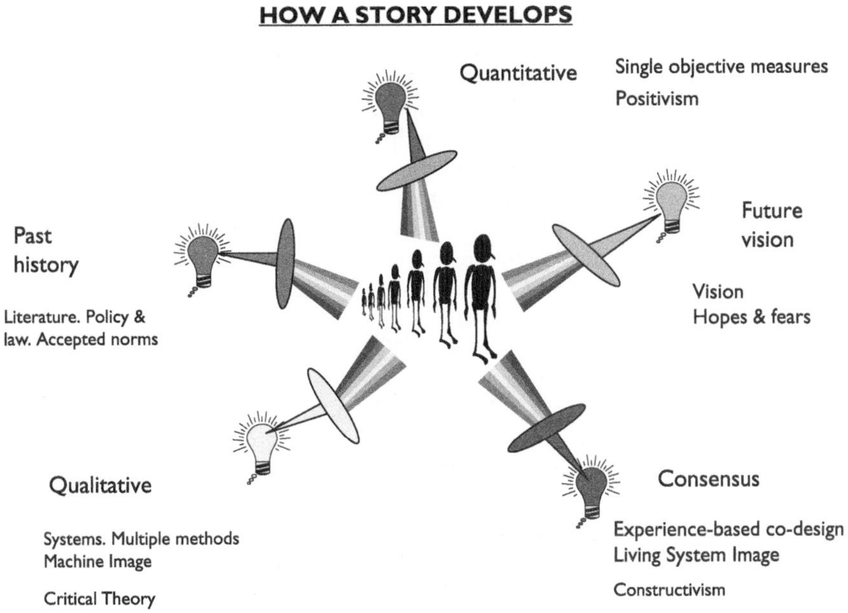

HOW A STORY DEVELOPS

Quantitative — Single objective measures / Positivism

Future vision — Vision / Hopes & fears

Past history — Literature. Policy & law. Accepted norms

Qualitative — Systems. Multiple methods / Machine Image / Critical Theory

Consensus — Experience-based co-design / Living System Image / Constructivism

Figure V Illuminating stories with complementary lenses

observing slow movement. What we 'see' depends on how we look, and what we are prepared to see.

The image challenges the value of any one way of looking. It highlights the value of multiple perspectives. Often, multiple-method evaluation is more insightful than a randomised controlled trial, stories more true than facts, community development more health-giving than individual treatments, shared leadership more effective than 'heroic' leaders.

Introduction to Part V: incremental transformations

> Most organisational theorists, as well as most philosophers, mistake the certainty of structures seen in hindsight for the emergent order that frames living forward. Neither group of scholars has come to grips with the fact that their conceptual understandings trail life and are of a different character than is living forward.
>
> (Soren Kierkegaard (1813–1855) re-phrased by
> Karl Weick, 1999)

Legend has it that Kierkegaard was so intolerant of those who imagined that the world is simple that when he died his brother used the funeral eulogy to apologise to all the people he had offended. 160 years later, a twenty-first-century leader of integrated care might empathise with the great man's frustration. Despite abundant evidence that co-creative leaps of imagination provide the spark to life that makes people feel healthy and fuel innovation, many people still expect linear, controlling behaviours to be sufficient. In research, we expect the randomised controlled trial to decide which model of integrated care is superior, yet we know that models need to adapt to the local context. In policy, we expect divisive markets and targets to cause efficiencies, yet we know that people give of their best when they feel part of a shared effort for quality. In development, we expect heroic individuals to lead improvements, yet we know that transformation of a whole system determines success.

Furthermore, these co-called 'linear thinkers' contradict themselves. They are managers who use only direct control with the people they work with, yet routinely use social media to experience the motivating power of community interaction. They are authors who claim that outcomes from an initiative happened in a linear way, then describe the non-linear journey they actually experienced. They are scientists who accept only quantitative research, yet they know that *love* does not plot on a bar graph. So 'linear thinkers' *do* use non-linear approaches when it suits them. It is not imagining the world to be simple that is the problem – it is imagining that it revolves around their way of thinking.

The same mistake often happens within relationships. Many are unable to see the co-constructive nature of a relationship and imagine that it revolves around them as individuals. They fail to realise that negotiation, appreciation and play are what are needed for success and see it as their job to directly control the other(s), often causing conflict, pain and poor performance, for themselves as well as for the relationship(s) as a whole.

Overly controlling behaviour can be caused by ignorance or selfishness – unable or unwilling to see beyond your own perspective. It can be caused by immaturity that prevents rising to the challenge of creatively interacting with others as equals. Some people don't know how to be equal or have a life script that tells them not to be. Some find it too challenging to believe that negotiation, learning and co-adaptation can produce better things than domination. *Individualism* inhibits many from valuing co-creative activities, and secular societies lack the habit of appreciating subtle interactions between hidden factors. These are some reasons why many find it too difficult to see beyond combat and control.

Many people *fear* emergence, anxious that they will not know what to do, or that things will spiral out of control, or that the process will reveal things they do not want to see – about the world or about themselves. They may not trust others to do things on their own. They may lack confidence in their own ability to steer things in productive directions.

This part shows how to take non-linear steps into a complex, unpredictable future without fear, by finding creative spaces within existing structures, playing good games and applying principles of organisational learning.

Vision, metaphors, theories, principles, methods

With one lens, community-oriented integrated care and health promotion (COIC) is a concrete fact – a well-oiled machine where each part does what it was designed for, according to a protocol. With a second lens, COIC is huge numbers of teams who work in interconnected silos where they develop their own languages and innovations. Look with a third lens and COIC is a dynamic process of ongoing co-adaptation, as people react to changing personalities, budgets, technology and health need; through this lens everyone is driven by a desire to make the whole thing work – everyone wants to 'sing in harmony'.

The third, *constructivist* lens is the one that sees processes of co-evolution that bind individuals, communities and networks together. This lens sees how people with different perspectives listen to each other and playfully interact to find a mutual accord – shared vision and shared stories. It sees how team players effortlessly interact with those they barely know to establish common purpose and co-create new ways of doing things.

Each of these three images of COIC has value. Each uses a different interpretation of vision, metaphor, theory, principles and methods. We can work with these to make COIC work.

A *vision* is: 'An image conjured up vividly in the imagination'. COIC has: 1) connected care pathways; 2) connected learning spaces; and 3) team players skilled at creative human interaction in both care pathways and connected learning spaces.

A *metaphor* is: 'An expression in which the thing referred to is described as if it really were what it merely represents'. COIC is: 1) a smooth running machine; 2) heroic entrepreneurs; and 3) Singing in harmony.

A *theory* is: 'A supposition or a system of ideas intended to explain something, especially one based on general principles independent of the thing to be explained'. COIC uses Darwin's theory of evolution that maintains that: 1) the world is an integrated whole; 2) each species is unique; 3) everything continually adapts to fit well with everything else.

A *principle* is: 'A fundamental truth or proposition that serves as the foundation for a system of belief or behaviour or for a chain of reasoning'. COIC needs: 1) organisations and systems that are fit for purpose; 2) practitioners that are fit for practice; and 3) networks of leadership teams that facilitate creative interaction and integrated working between individuals, organisations and systems.

A *method* is: 'A particular procedure for accomplishing or approaching something, especially a systematic or established one'. COIC needs: 1) care quality commission assessment of the fitness of organisations; 2) revalidation to assess the fitness of individual practitioners; and 3) an applied research unit that organises team-building workshops to help different teams to fit well together.

Chapter 17

Networks for complicated journeys

Key message: Community-oriented integrated care is a social movement and a machine.

In this chapter:

- Social network theory
- A railway network allows functional and transformational activities
- Social network theory again
- Relevance of social network theory to community-oriented integrated care

Social network theory

The previous part (IV) shows that *community-oriented integrated care* (COIC) cannot be described with one lens or image or theory. It is, at the same time, a machine that treats diseases and a social movement for whole-society health. It is a mechanism that facilitates shared care for those who are sick and inter-organisational collaboration for ongoing health improvements. It enables functional and transformational activities at the same time.

Social network theory helps to imagine combined functional and transformational activities within COIC.

Social network theory tells us that:

A *network* is: 'a set of nodes and the set of ties representing some relationship, or lack of relationship, between the nodes'.

Nodes are: 'people, places or organisations that enable multidisciplinary transfer of information, broker partnerships for quality improvements, and access a variety of resources and power. They are places where different paths converge, and the means whereby a network reaches places that bureaucratic structures cannot reach.'

Ties are: 'relationships between network members and manifest as cross organisational partnerships, committee meetings and multidisciplinary teams'.

Density is: 'the number of ties in the network in proportion to the number of possible ties'.

Centralisation is: 'the degree to which different members are central or peripheral to power and refers to the mechanisms of policy formation, including executive management groups, formal and informal leaders, think-tanks, and ways that intelligence throughout the network influences overall direction'.

Thomas, P., Graffy, J., Wallace, P. and Kirby, M. How primary care networks can help integrate academic and service initiatives in primary care. *The Annals of Family Medicine*, 2006, 4: 235–239

One question is: *what nodes, ties and centralisation help people to navigate healthcare systems in ways that enhance health and care, and also continually improve the quality of the whole system?* One way to approach this question is to consider the transferable lessons from a familiar network – a railway network.

A railway network allows functional and transformational activities

Imagine that you want to use a railway network. You want to undertake complicated activities like travelling to different destinations, and also complex activities like developing relationships with new people. What will help you to achieve these twin goals?

- **Reliable maps and timetables:** These help to explore new destinations. Imagine a railway network that does not have route maps – this would make it difficult to plan even one trip, let alone a complicated journey.
- **Enjoyable ways to get to know fellow passengers:** Imagine a journey that is full of hostile people; and another that is full of interesting, friendly people who you can easily talk with. Which is more likely to motivate people to travel?
- **Easy ways to change routes:** Imagine a train line that has no stations where you can change trains – you would not be able to take complicated journeys.
- **Evaluation:** Imagine a railway network that does not audit whether the trains run on time, or fails to notice changing passenger demand, or does not listen to complaints. Would you trust it?

In integrated care, both patients and practitioners are 'travellers'. Both need to navigate the whole system. Both need to work with others for shared care. Both need to contribute to improvement of the system. As in a railway network, they need system maps and timetables, enjoyable encounters, opportunities to improve things, and data to see what is going on.

Social network theory again

Nodes

In community-oriented integrated care and health promotion (COIC) nodes are people, places or organisations that refer into care pathways and collaborate for care and health promotion. In the UK, these are general practices, community services, intermediate care, hospitals, local authorities, public health, schools, third-sector organisations and others.

Integrated care needs a description of what each node does and where it is.

Ties and density of ties

For functional activities, like referring patients for specialist care, integrated care needs large numbers of linear ties – care pathway for every kind of disease. For transformational activities, like building trusted relationships throughout a system, it needs a small number of complex ties – information-rich people from different parts of the system interact to share ideas and envision ways to improve things.

COIC needs maps that show how the nodes connect for functional activities (e.g. referrals) and timetables for multidisciplinary events like co-designing system-wide improvements.

Centralisation

For complicated activities, like implementing policy, integrated care needs top-down direction, rewards, sanctions and markers of progress. For complex activities, like working out what that policy should be, it needs *connected learning spaces* where stakeholders can crystallise meaning from experience and evidence.

COIC needs annual cycles of inter-organisational learning and change that allow top-down and co-creative activities to be intertwined.

Relevance of social network theory to community-oriented integrated care

The most obvious insight from social network theory for COIC is the need for maps that show how different things connect. This includes directories of resources, care pathways and decision support. On the other hand, social network theory also shows the need for people in different parts of the system to routinely interact in ways that facilitate or stimulate improvements of the whole system and good traveller experiences.

As with a railway network, COIC needs to show how and where to engage:

- **Local health communities:** Just as railway networks need stations where different routes connect and people can get to know each other, COIC needs geographic areas where care pathways connect and people co-develop local health communities
- **Shared care for long-term conditions:** Just as frequent travellers have season tickets to travel on certain trains, patients with long-term conditions have care plans that describe the care pathways they may benefit from using.
- **Seasons of care, health promotion and participatory action research:** Just as a train company regularly reviews what is needed at different times of year through customer feedback and strategic planning, health care needs to review its operation through annual cycles of learning and change, and routinely gathered data.
- **Infrastructure of facilitation and communication:** Just as train companies develop staff, repair trains and provide intelligence of what is happening, COIC needs training, problem solving and data that support continuous quality improvements.

Community-oriented integrated care is much more complicated than a railway network. Large numbers of practitioners and managers undertake vast a number of different kinds of actions every day. Social network theory shows how to design infrastructure for them to achieve these different things in mutually enhancing ways.

Social network theory helps us to see how to design systems that facilitate healthy human interaction as well as control movements of large numbers of people. Combined facilitation and control can be stimulated by imaginative policy. For example, people can *compete* to lead *collaborative* projects. Agreements can be *negotiated*, then *policed*. People can be advised what to do *and* helped to think for themselves. People can be assessed for their competence as individuals *and* as team players.

Network theory helps to design connections in a system. Techniques such as systems mapping and backwards mapping (Chapter 7) help to see glitches in those systems, ways to improve them, and where data need to be gathered to understand what is going on.

Social network theory helps to design the architecture for different people to encounter others. It does not reveal how people should interact in such encounters. That is the subject of the next chapter.

Chapter 18

Developing team players and systems thinkers

Key message: Everyone needs to be a team player and a systems-thinker.

In this chapter:

- Integrated care is a network of teams
- The history of teams in health care
- Integrated care needs more than teams – it needs team players
- Team players play three different roles in 'music'
- Common sense

    o stimulates complex interactions
    o helps people to travel hopefully
    o leads to incremental transformations
    o disappears at a distance

- People play games to develop relationships
- People need to play good games to develop healthy relationships
- Becoming trapped in one ego state prevents healthy relationships
- Relevance of transactional analysis to community-oriented integrated care

Integrated care is a network of teams

You can get things done when both you and the people you are communicating listen well to each other and adapt to enhance each other, making your combined efforts more than the sum of the parts. This is what high-performing teams do. Rugby players see the cues that team members give in their words and their body language, they anticipate new patterns and try out a new move, trusting the others to respond creatively – so the team acts 'as one'.

Community-oriented integrated care (COIC) can be thought of as a complex network of teams. Here are examples of interventions that systematically developed networks of teams to enhance integrated working (also described in Chapter 13):

- Lambert's *team-building workshop programme* developed multidisciplinary primary care teams, supported by local organising teams made up of middle managers from the health authority and partner organisations.

- The King's Fund *whole-system initiatives* recruited people from all parts of a city into teams that facilitated change across multiple organisational boundaries.
- Ashton's *new public health* combined primary care and public health leadership to support local communities.
- Liverpool's *local multidisciplinary facilitation teams* facilitated collaboration between general practices, public health, universities, health authorities, trade unions and voluntary groups in geographic areas of 70,000 population.
- Mead's *community development agencies* engaged whole populations in seeing health as '*a citizen issue, not a medical issue*'.
- De Koning's *participatory research* built communities for health improvement in developing countries.

The history of teams in health care

The term 'team' in old English means family or company. In farming, it described a team of oxen harnessed together. The modern sense of 'persons associated in some joint action' comes from the 1520s, 'team player' from 1886, 'team spirit' from 1928.

Recognition that health care needs multidisciplinary teams is relatively new. Heinemann and Zeiss analysed evaluation instruments for team working in health-care settings, and provided a useful summary of the history of team-working in health care in the USA:

> As medical specialties developed in the early 1900s, physicians viewed the team approach as a mechanism for coordinating the medical specialties ... In the 1930s, nurses began to advocate for the team approach in hospital settings as a means of coordinating the efforts of growing numbers of health professionals in health workers employed there. By the mid-1900s, teams were providing care to chronically ill patients in such areas as home care, mental health, and rehabilitation. President Johnson's Great Society and War on Poverty Programs of the 1960s gave impetus to teamwork delivered in community-based, primary care settings to poor and underserved, urban populations ... in the 21st-century, a team approach to health care is continuing to enjoy favour as a result of restructuring of health care organisations analogous to businesses.
>
> (Heinemann and Zeiss, 2002)

 Heinemann, G.D. and Zeiss, A.M. *Team Performance in Healthcare: Assessment and Development*. New York: Kluwer Academic/Plenum Publishers, 2002

The authors drew on two theoretical frameworks to create a model of team performance: 1) stages of small group development and 2) teams embedded within larger organisations. They analysed team function by a) structure, b) context, c) process and d) productivity.

Working with the 12 directors of the Veterans Affairs (VA) Inter-professional Team Training and Development (ITTD) programme, they identified different kinds of teams – management teams that set policy and provide organisational leadership, inter-professional clinical teams and natural work groups. They were responsible for one or more specific functions within a health-care organisation, and short-term quality improvement teams, committees, and task forces that organised around specific issues.

The authors reviewed 53 instruments that assess and develop teams in different health-care contexts, and categorised then by their ability to address more than one domain:

- 11 focused instruments, e.g. attitudes towards health-care teams
- 11 middle-range instruments, e.g. team integration measure
- 15 broad spectrum instruments, e.g. team climate inventory
- 16 full spectrum instruments, e.g. team effectiveness profile

Of these, they identified 22 instruments that were being used, or had the potential to be used by health-care teams.

The work was of high quality. It was methodical and insightful and involved some of the most knowledgeable people in the area. It was a labour of love.

Integrated care needs more than teams – it needs team players

One confronting thing about the Heinemann and Zeiss analysis is that not one of their 53 instruments is adequate for community-oriented integrated care as envisioned here. All the instruments assume that teams are relatively unchanging, have regular meetings and develop plans for patients care (p. 360). Health care does need such teams. But they are not enough for integrated care and integrated health promotion.

Integrated care of the future requires a more dynamic understanding of team. Everyone needs to be a *team player*, able to attend just one meeting and make a valuable contribution; able to belong to dozens of teams in virtual ways; able to know how to systematically build trusted relationships with different kinds of people in different contexts. Health-care teams of the future need to do more than patient care; they also need to contribute to networks of teams for leadership, innovation, evaluated improvements and more.

Chapter 15 explains that the constantly changing nature of the world means that to be healthy and to take a confident role in integrated care, individuals need to be able to:

1   Be alive in the moment
2   Adventure optimistically in an uncertain world
3   Be a team player
4   Be a life-long, life-wide learner
5   Be resilient

The kind of team player needed by community-oriented integrated care has these life skills in abundance. He or she is an action learner, action researcher, boundary-spanning, systems-thinker who listens deeply, appreciates others, and is skilled at techniques to get the best out of difficulties and pursue a vision for whole-person, whole-family, whole-community health.

We need team players with high-level skills. They can finish off each other's sentences and take intuitive collective actions that succeed as though by magic. They can role-play different perspectives, lead and observe with equal comfort. They give a sense that no mountain is too high to climb, every situation has opportunities and no adversity is too big to rise above. And then they make effective plans. Not everyone has this potential. Some are born with these skills, but most of us have to painstakingly develop them through years of practice.

We need new instruments to evaluate team players.

Team players play three different roles in 'music'

Team players need to be able to switch between three different types of interaction with other team members that reflect Guba's three paradigms of inquiry (Chapter 16). These can be likened to three different responsibilities when playing music:

- **Scripted music:** Team members have to 'play' exactly the notes given to them; for example protocols for long-term conditions or delivering reports on time. Like an orchestra or a military band this kind of activity needs to be delivered exactly as the script dictates. The script is the thing that leads them to do exactly what is needed.
- **Soloists:** Team members have to 'play' on their own; for example a receptionist welcomes a patient, a manager gives a talk, a clinician consults. They have elbow room to be creative but they must be mindful of the rest of the 'band' – keeping eye contact, recognising when others can join in, deferring to skills, referring and appreciating the whole 'tune'. The conductor leads them to come in at the right time.
- **Jazz:** Health-care teams need to creatively 'play' together; for example co-creating a care plan, devising a pilot project or responding to someone's emotional needs. Like a jazz band, team members need to cleverly *play off each other*. Unlike scripted and solo 'playing', this type of *play* is closer to its common usage – a game between people, especially children. Leadership for this type of music is *shared* – they take it in turns and do it in synchrony.

As team players we need to move between following the script, following the conductor and following our instincts, in ways that are appropriate to the needs of the moment. Playing 'music' with team members develops us as team players as well as produces good outcomes. Not everyone needs to be a highly skilled 'musician', but everyone needs at least basic skills in contributing in these three different ways.

PAUSE: How do you develop team skills in yourself and in others?

Common sense stimulates complex interactions

A mother and child walked to the park. She said: 'A car is coming, move quickly onto the pavement' . . . 'Which way shall we go to the swings?' . . . 'Look, your friends, let's forget the swings and play with them.'

In these three everyday sentences, she stimulated three very different kinds of interaction.

- The first sentence is direct and controlling – a 'simple' situation where fast, direct action is needed. The mother assumes control. This is a parent–child interaction.

- The second sentence is mindful of different perspectives – a 'complicated' situation where the best action is not immediately clear. Both actors consider different options and negotiate the best for their purposes. This is an adult–adult transaction.
- The third sentence is exploratory and creative – an emergent 'complex' situation where the intention is not to solve a problem but to open out new possibilities. This involves *play* to co-create new things. This is a child–child transaction.

Without thinking about it, both mother and child felt it natural to switch between these different types of interaction to respond to their changing context; and they happened within seconds of each other. It resulted in a shared story about their visit to the park.

You can see these three types of interaction in high-performing teams in health care – for example in a resuscitation team called to someone who has had a cardiac arrest. When urgent direct action is needed, you will see someone assume control and tell the others what to do – 'Adrenaline!' 'Stand Back!' 'Shock!' When there are different options for the next steps, for example whether to transfer to another place, you will see thoughtful sharing of knowledge and discussion about the best thing to do. When the situation is under control, you will see exploration of new potential that looks like playful banter – 'Interesting meeting last week'; 'Lots of traffic today'; 'What are you doing tonight?'

Team players need to be able to quickly move between these three kinds of interaction. Using too much of one kind results in unhealthy relationships. The first enables fast direct action; too much leads to a controlling, dependent relationship. The second considers the complications in a situation; too much leads to an intense, cerebral relationship. The third explores new ways of doing things; too much leads to a fickle, irresponsible relationship. A dynamic, co-creative combination of all three is the secret of a healthy relationship. It is common sense.

Common sense helps people to travel hopefully

Perhaps because we use it all the time, it is easy to forget how sophisticated 'common sense' is. It involves subconscious recognition of opportunities to move a story on in a healthy way. Second by second, we react to what we hear, see and feel. Common sense involves *active listening* – to ourselves as well as to those around us, and to the broad range of *whispers* that help us to glimpse so much more. Checking out with others the sense they make of this array of information is where the term comes from; we discuss a situation to make sense of it – to achieve 'sense-held-in-common', con-sensus, com-mon sense.

Chapter 15 explains that good health means more than lying back and reminiscing a coherent, positive past life story. It means developing my story into the future by creatively interacting in the world. This means adventures that help my story to develop in new and valuable ways that enrich my sense of narrative unity. This requires me to *travel hopefully*. This is also common sense – we all know that staying the same leads to stagnation. Moving on, with hope in our hearts and a 'can-do' attitude is a good formula for success.

Common sense also tells us that transformational change is slow, yet actions to achieve it can involve sudden, timely interventions. Common sense tells us to be patient, listen carefully to others and think strategically. And also be alert – be ready to pounce.

Common sense helps me to tell if my story is evolving in a hopeful direction or not. If the actors on my present stage behave in ways that make me believe that our shared story is evolving in mutually enhancing and positive ways, things are probably heading in a healthy direction. If not, I might be better to look for another stage. But I must be patient and look deep – things that make no sense on the surface may be full of meaning at other levels.

Common sense leads to incremental transformations

The three types of interaction – parent–child; adult–adult; child–child – are the transactional equivalents of Guba's three inquiry paradigms: 1) parent–child, like positivism, is concerned with linear, focused interactions, and is used to control others; 2) adult–adult, like critical theory, is concerned with understanding different perspectives and is used to consider different options; 3) child–child, like constructivism, is concerned with co-creating new opportunities, and is used to bind people together. Each has strengths and weaknesses. In combination, they provide the basic tools to move forward our life stories.

The third kind of interaction – child–child – binds people together through *games* to which each makes a different but equal contribution. Participants co-create a fun, shared story. It weaves different coloured threads into a tapestry. It turns 'I' into 'we'. *Play* is the magic ingredient. It is the source of creativity and fun. You can tell it is happening because participants laugh together, and good things happen.

When these three kinds of interaction are used skilfully, they incrementally transform stories. *Skilfully* is key. Each player will be playing a different 'tune', to a different 'beat' that is their life story. If you are 'in tune' with others you can co-create beautiful music. If not you create discord. Changing your 'beat' to be compatible means letting go of part of your identity – uncomfortable. However, when you have mastered a new beat that works, you will find that your old tune fits into it more beautifully than ever before – it will be transformed into a new beat. The difficulty is that you have to let it go to get it back. Not everyone is ready to do this.

The mother and the child going for a walk in the park show that incremental transformations are everyday activities. Thousands of everyday interactions like this can, over time, transform health care from silo-thinking into team-thinking.

Common sense disappears at a distance

Common sense disappears at a distance. When the context drifts out of view, its multiple subtle nuances go with it. When people observe rather than participate, they do not feel the experience in the same way. This poses a dilemma to those who have to manage and lead large numbers of people within integrated care – how much do you tell people what to do, and how much do you let them work it out for themselves?

Some managers only use 'top-down' micro-control – they tell the 'mother' what to do. Others only use a 'bottom-up' style that leaves the 'mother' to find her own way. Both can be useful at times, but neither on its own is enough because they both separate manager and 'mother', so they do not share the emerging story. Instead, managers should dip in and out of the situation, playing and negotiating as well as controlling and leaving alone.

To develop as team players people need everyday opportunities to switch between modes of interaction – controlling, facilitating, playing, leaving alone. They need to interact with others to share stories, envision new ways of doing things, and have shared adventures. This is pretty much what mother's groups do – stories shared over cups of tea about their walks in the park, sharing ideas about new kinds of walk and then going on those walks together.

And they laugh and they smile. Because they are playing 'good games'.

People play games to develop relationships

In his theory of transactional analysis, Berne describes *parent, adult* and *child* as three *ego states* that people move in and out of, when having conversations. He describes rules of interaction that lead to acceptable communication. *Crossed transactions* feel disrespectful and un-listening, and break off communication. So if someone speaks with parent–child mode, the responder needs to reply in child–parent mode, before switching to another transaction type. Sequences of such transactions build up what Berne calls 'games'.

Ego states as described by Berne use more than *spoken* language. He writes:

> from time to time people show noticeable changes in posture, view-point, voice, vocabulary, and other aspects of behaviour. In a given individual, a certain set of behaviour patterns corresponds to one state of mind, while another set is related to a different psychic attitude, often inconsistent with the first.

(p. 24)

 Berne, E. *Games People Play: the psychology of human relationships*. London: Penguin, 1964

Ego states are the same kind of thing as 'mental models', 'lenses' and 'mindsets' described elsewhere in this book. Each is a 'world of being' that includes ways of thinking, seeing and acting, assumptions about what to expect from others, and what to expect from myself. They bring facial expressions, language, tone of voice. You can put them on and take them off like a coat. When their use fits the context, as with the mother and the child in the park, they feel natural and mutually enhancing. When they don't, they feel manipulative and controlling.

Team players need to be highly skilled at healthy interactions. It involves deep listening, respect for difference and mental agility. They need to respond to others as expected, then shift to a different transaction mode that develops a 'good game'. So if a conversation stops after a mother says 'A car is coming, move quickly onto the pavement' (parent–child), the game might be called 'I'm in charge'. A skilled team player might say 'Thank you, Mummy' (child–parent), then 'You know I had already seen the car' (adult–adult), or 'I really enjoy our walks' (child–child). The 'child' had shifted the trajectory of exchanges to a game that might (if the mother also plays well) be called 'We are equals, and we are mates'.

Berne describes procedures, rituals, pastimes and games as a 'series of programmed transactions' that make up conversations:

- 'Procedures' – 'a series of simple complementary adult transactions directed towards the manipulation of reality'; for example, agreeing actions for a care plan
- 'Rituals' – 'a stereotyped series of simple complementary transactions programmed by external social forces'; for example, a 'huddle' where a team stands in a circle to briefly discuss the day's work
- 'Pastimes' – 'a series of semi-ritualistic, simple, complementary transactions, arranged around a single field of material, whose primary object is to structure an interval of time'; for example, 'catching up' at lunch breaks
- 'Games' – 'an ongoing series of complementary ulterior transactions, progressing to well-defined predictable outcome'; for example, 'Why don't you . . . Yes, but'

Procedures, rituals, pastimes and games all help to build relationships and teams.

People need to play good games to develop healthy relationships

Like everyone else, Berne is bound by his context. Not many people go to a psychiatrist complaining that their relationships are too good! Consequently he describes how people use games in harmful, divisive ways. He states: 'Many games are played most intensely by disturbed people; generally speaking, the more disturbed they are, the harder they play.'

Berne describes 12 categories that include 36 'bad games', and a meagre five 'good games' (for example 'Happy to Help').

Thomas Harris went the other way. He proposed playing 'good games' to make everyday life fun and productive. He uses transactional analysis to purposefully stimulate healthy relationships and healthy cultures. He wrote:

> Transactional analysis . . . is a teaching and learning device . . . If the relationships between two people can be made creative, fulfilling, and free from fear, then it follows that this can work for two relationships, or three or one hundred or, we are convinced, for relationships that affect entire social groups, even nations.

(p. xvii)

 Harris, T.A. *I'm OK – You're OK.* Reading: Arrow Books, 1995

So, 'good games' help us to grow in healthy ways and build healthy relationships. Team players in health care need to play 'good games'. As Harris might have said: 'You are OK. Actually I am OK too. We are different, very different. But we are both OK. Let's play.'

People are not usually conscious of the games they play; nor of their power to both hurt and to heal others. The 'glass half-empty' person is unaware of the misery they cause to others by always finding fault. The 'glass half-full' person is unaware of the motivation they give to others by combining optimism with thoughtful assessment.

Acknowledging the games that we habitually play is necessary for personal transformation. To recognise them we must surface what Argyris and Schon call 'theories-in-use' – the hidden beliefs that guide our actions. These are quite different from our espoused theories – what we say we believe. When hidden beliefs are visible, we can do something about them.

Becoming trapped in one ego state prevents healthy relationships

Berne describes the immaturity of those who exhibit a constant 'ego state'. He caricatures professions that might do this as a way of life:

- Parent – uniformly judgemental; e.g. a clergyman
- Adult – fun-less, objective scientist; e.g. a diagnostician
- Child – 'little old me'; e.g. clowns

 Berne, E. *Transactional Analysis in Psychotherapy: the classic handbook to its principles*. London: Souvenir Press, 1991 (p. 35)

People who are stuck in one ego state are poor at developing themselves and their relationships because they lack ability to play good games that can change their story-lines. They repeat the same tune. Without adaptation there can be no novelty, no surprise, no fun. Their relationships are one dimensional and are boring except to those who also enjoy this dimension of interaction. Someone who is stuck in one ego state is likely to dismiss others as being inferior and distance himself or herself from them, inevitably creating boundaries, walls, conflict, fragmentation. Such a person is stuck in an 'I–It' mindset (Chapter 15).

A healthy person needs a more sophisticated way of thinking.

Relevance of transactional analysis to community-oriented integrated care

Berne's transactional analysis shows how to build trusted relationships and team players through everyday encounters. Team players use Berne's procedures, rituals and pastimes to provide everyday opportunities to encourage healthy interactions. They use 'good games' to build trusted relationships and high-performing teams.

'Good games' bring a spark of life into otherwise cold interactions; a breath of fresh air into heavy conversations; a cheeky smile into an otherwise stiff face. They motivate people to higher levels of operation; they enable innovative solutions. They make everyone feel 'OK'.

Merely being mindful of the need to play good games may be all someone needs to start to build the trusted relationships they need for a healthy, happy life. It is certainly a good start.

Chapter 19

Learning organisations build teams, communities and systems

Key message: Organisations and systems as well as individuals need to continually learn and change.

In this chapter:

* The learning organisation story

    o   Lewin
    o   Freire
    o   Brown and Duguid

* Definitions of a learning organisation

    o   Mike Pedlar, Tom Boydell and John Burgoyne
    o   Andrew Mayo and Elizabeth Lank
    o   Nancy Dixon
    o   Peter Senge

* Key characteristics of a learning organisation

    o   Chris Argyris and Donald Schon's three types of learning
    o   The Social Care Institute for Excellence 2004 resource pack
    o   Peter Senge's fifth discipline – systems thinking
    o   Work-based learning

* Kolb's learning cycle
* Learning organisations in the NHS
* Relevance of organisational learning to community-oriented integrated care

The learning organisation story

Learning is, in its essence, a fundamentally social phenomenon.

 Wenger, E (1998) *Communities of Practice: learning, meaning, and identity.* Cambridge: Cambridge University Press (p. 3)

Wenger explains that *learning organisations* expect learning to be more than the accumulation of knowledge. Organisational members learn from and with each other, as a way of life. This chapter describes some of the stages in the learning organisation story.

Kurt Lewin (1890–1947), a German-American psychologist, pioneered organisational, social and applied psychology. He suggested that neither nature (inborn tendencies) nor nurture (how life experiences shape individuals) alone can account for individuals' behaviour and personalities; instead, both nature and nurture interact to shape each person. He called this *field theory*. Lewin recognised that the world is much more complicated than it appears at first sight and change requires an understanding of human interaction and power as well as individual actions. This led to his famous quote: 'If you want to truly understand something, try to change it.' Lewin coined the terms 'action research', 'force field analysis', and 'group dynamics'. He explained that organisations should periodically 'unfreeze' – renew vision and strategy; then 'freeze' – focus on getting jobs done, before the next time to unfreeze.

 Lewin, K. *Resolving Social Conflicts: field theory in social science. Selected Papers.* Washington: American Psychological Association, 1997

Paulo Freire, writing in the late 1960s, challenged the relevance of learning as accumulation of facts, which he called the 'banking concept of learning'. He emphasised learning from real-life situations. He described a need for *critical consciousness* to empower people to act on learning in synchronised ways. He maintained that the banking concept of learning *actually oppresses people* by setting those with theoretical knowledge above others. In contrast, 'problem posing education . . . affirms men and women as beings in the process of becoming . . . It roots itself in the dynamic present and becomes revolutionary' (p. 84)

 Freire, P. *Pedagogy of the Oppressed.* New York: Continuum, 2003

John Brown and Paul Duguid develop Freire's argument that true learning is applied, and in its application, participants build communities of practice:

> [past theories of] training [have been] thought of as the transmission of explicit, abstract knowledge from the head of someone who knows to the head of someone who does not, in surroundings that specifically exclude the complexities of practice and the communities of practitioners. The setting for learning is simply assumed not to matter . . .
>
> . . . concepts of knowledge or information transfer, however, have been under increasing attack in recent years . . . What is learned is profoundly connected to the conditions in which it was learned . . .
>
> . . . learners do not receive or even construct abstract, objective, individual knowledge; rather they learn to function in the community . . . They acquire that particular community's subjective viewpoint and learn to speak its language. In short, they are enculturated . . .
>
> . . . workplace learning is best understood, then, in terms of the communities being formed or joined and personal identities being changed. The essential issue in learning is becoming a practitioner, not learning about practice.
>
> (pp. 68–69)

 Brown, J.S. and Duguid, P. Organisational learning and communities of practice: toward a unified view of working, learning, and innovation. In Cohen, M.D. and Sproull, L.S. (eds) *Organisational Learning.* Thousand Oaks, CA: Sage, 1996, pp. 58–82

Definitions of a learning organisation

Forrest lists four complementary definitions of a learning organisation (p. ix):

Mike Pedlar, Tom Boydell and John Burgoyne:

- An organisation which facilitates the learning of all its members and continually transforms itself

Andrew Mayo and Elizabeth Lank:

- A learning organisation harnesses the full brainpower, knowledge and experience available to it, in order to evolve continually for the benefit of all its stakeholders

Nancy Dixon:

- A learning organisation is one which intentionally uses learning processes at individual, group and system level to continuously transform the organisation in a direction that is increasingly satisfying to its stakeholders

Peter Senge:

- An organisation which is continually expanding its capacity to create its own future

 Forrest, A. *Fifty Ways Towards a Learning Organisation.* Dover: The Industrial Society, 1999

Key characteristics of a learning organisation

Chris Argyris and Donald Schon's three types of learning

Responding in 1996 to criticism of learning organisation theory, Argyris and Schon distinguished between the literature of 'the learning organisation' and the scholarly literature of 'organisational learning'. They wrote:

> The learning organisation literature includes notions of organisational adaptability, flexibility, avoidance of stability traps, propensity to experiment, readiness to rethink means and ends, inquiry-orientation, realisation of human potential for learning in the service of organisational processes, and creation of organisational settings as context for human development.
>
> (p. 180)

> The *organisational learning* literature focuses on just those questions the first branch ignores: What does organisational learning mean? How is organisational learning at all feasible? What kind of organisational learning is desirable, and for whom and with what chance of actually occurrence? The scholars of organisational learning generally adopt a sceptical stance towards these questions.
>
> (p. 188)

> proponents of the learning organisation are not worried about the meaningfulness of organisational learning and take its desirability to be axiomatic. (p.198) . . .

The problems raised by two branches of the literature are largely complementary: what one branch treats as centrally important, the other tends to ignore. Both branches do concern themselves with the capability of real-world organisations to draw valid and useful inferences from experience and observation and to convert such inferences to effective action.

(p. 199)

They describe three types of productive organisational learning (pp. 20–29):

1   **Single-loop learning:** Instrumental learning clarifies facts. It focuses on how to improve the status quo. It involves incremental change and narrows the gaps between desired and actual conditions. Single loop learning is the most prevalent form of learning in organisations.
2   **Double-loop learning:** Surfaces and changes hidden and interconnected factors. It focuses on how to change the status quo. Members learn how to change the existing assumptions and conditions within which single-loop learning operates.
3   **Deutero-learning:** Learning how to learn. Learning is directed at the learning process itself and uses interaction of ideas to improve both single- and double-loop learning.

 Argyris, C. and Schon, D. *Organisational Learning II: theory, methods and practice*. Reading, MA: Addison-Wesley, 1996

Here is yet another example of Guba's three paradigms (Chapter 16) being rediscovered by others: single loop = simple; double loop = complicated; deutero-learning = complex.

The Social Care Institute for Excellence 2004 resource pack

This resource lists key characteristics of learning organisations:

- Management that enhance opportunities for employee, carer and service user involvement in the organisation
- A culture of openness, creativity and experimentation
- Service-user and carer feedback and participation is actively sought
- Cross-organisational and collaborative working
- Effective information systems for both internal and external communication
- Informed decision-making including the involvement of relevant local people in decision-making (e.g. social care workers and managers, and users)
- Critical appraisal skills, peer support and appropriate supervision, learning from mistakes and sharing knowledge
- A learning environment that encourages the exploration of new ideas
- Team-working and team-learning
- Leaders who model openness, risk-taking and reflection, and communicate a compelling vision of the learning organisation

 Learning Organisations: a self-assessment resources pack. London: Social Care Institute for Excellence, 2004

Peter Senge's fifth discipline – systems thinking

Senge described five disciplines of a learning organisation. The *fifth discipline* is the one that binds them – system's thinking.

1   Personal mastery – the discipline of personal growth and learning
2   Mental models – the way you think determines the way you behave
3   Building shared vision – co-creating collaborative force of impressive power
4   Team learning – like a great jazz band, feeding off each other's creativity
5   Systems thinking – sees connections between different things

 Senge, P. *The Fifth Discipline: the art and science of the learning organization.* London: Random House, 1999

Work-based learning

Work-based learning is routine in learning organisations. People learn from their everyday work. In general practice, this includes reflection on patient encounters, team-learning, case studies, significant events, and whole-organisation workshops and team exercises.

Work-based learning includes experiential learning. This means more than simply accumulating facts from daily experience. It also means reflection – reflecting what you experience against what you think you know, to check if they are in accord. When there is a mismatch, you ask more questions and listen more deeply until it makes sense. Then you have truly learned.

Partnership between clinical commissioning groups and academic institutions can use work-based learning to develop leaders for integrated care. Leadership teams can bring their improvement projects to a leadership course and use them to learn from and with each other, at the same time improving the impact of their work. Such courses need to be part of the infrastructure for community-oriented integrated care (Part I), supporting leadership of collaboration and integration from general practices (Part II) and from geographic localities (Part III).

Kolb's learning cycle

David Kolb, whose experiential learning model underpins modern thinking about how individuals learn, wrote in 1996 how the model can be applied to organisations. His model contains two poles (concrete experience v. abstract conceptualisation, and active experimentation v. reflective observation); together they provide four stages in a repeatable cycle of learning: 1) observations and reflections; 2) formation of abstract concepts and generalisations; 3) testing implications in new situations; 4) concrete experience.

Kolb explained that different people tend to be more or less strong at different stages of the cycle. Some roles need these strengths, so they naturally attract people who are strong in those stages. This can give a misleading impression that the other stages are less important. He described his *learning style inventory* that helps individuals to analyse their strengths in each stage as a way to build teams that are strong in all four stages. He explained that specialisation might help short-term success, but in the long term it can reduce effectiveness through reduced ability to learn and change. He concludes:

> The nature of the learning process is such that [these] opposing perspectives - action and reflection, concrete involvement and analytical detachment - are essential for optimal learning. When one perspective comes to dominate others, learning effectiveness is reduced in the long run. From this we can conclude that the most effective learning systems are those that can tolerate differences in perspective.

 Kolb, D. Management and the learning process. In Starkey, K. (ed.) *How Organisations Learn*. London: International Thomson Publishing, 1996, pp. 270–287

Kolb reminds us that cycles of learning and change need to continue forever, both for individuals and for organisations. Cycles of single-loop, double-loop and deutero-learning are all needed. Learners *do* need to clarify facts, but they also need to understand connections, and they need to continually increase their capacity to learn and change.

These theorists all emphasise that within these cycles of learning participants need to be able to (gently) challenge each other. Charles Handy similarly emphasised the importance of challenge from different perspectives. He wrote:

> provided it did not degenerate into conflict . . . differences are essential to change. If there were no urge to compete and no need to disagree the organisation would be either in a state of apathy or of complacency – both triggers of decline in a constantly changing world.
>
> (pp. 318, 313)

 Handy, C. *Understanding Organisations*. London: Penguin, 1993

Learning organisations in the NHS

In 2001, Valerie Iles and Kim Sutherland reviewed the evidence in the field of change management with the intention of informing change in the NHS. They listed a range of techniques to understand complexity and analyse what can be changed. Then they listed four ways to make change happen:

1   Organisational development
2   Organisational learning and the learning organisation
3   Action research
4   Project management

They noted that, despite interest, there has been no documented example of adopting and evaluating the organisational learning/learning organisations idea at scale:

> The concept of the Learning Organisation is increasingly popular as organisations, subjected to exhortations to become more adaptable and responsive to change, attempt to develop structures and systems that nurture innovation . . .

There is little hard evidence of the effect of organisational learning in practice. Argyris and Schon states (1996) that they are unaware of any organisation that has fully implemented a double-loop learning system . . .

In the context of health, there are a handful of articles that discuss issues surrounding the use of organisational learning in the NHS but no empirical or evaluative reports.

(p. 65)

 Iles, V. and Sutherland, K. *Managing Change in the NHS. Organisational change: a review for health care managers, professionals and researchers*. London: London School of Hygiene and Tropical Medicine, 2001

Relevance of organisational learning to community-oriented integrated care

Through their ability to integrate teams, build communities and develop individuals as team players, *learning organisations* are important for integrated care. Healthcare organisations, networks and communities, including general practices, should routinely practise Senge's five disciplines and Argyris and Shon's three types of learning. They should develop staff as 'systems thinkers' who habitually oscillate their attention between focused detail and 'bigger pictures'. They should engage in ongoing cycles of inter-organisational learning and change.

Parts I, II and III describe ways to do this, through policy (Part I), through locally based organisations (Part II) and from geographic areas (Part III).

There is an urgent need to address Iles and Sutherland's criticism and evaluate case studies of organisational learning to provide evidence of their effect. Routinely gathering data should be aligned to such case studies to evidence the overall effects of multiple initiatives.

Chapter 20

Public health and primary care – an essential partnership

Key message: All citizens need to contribute to a healthy world.

In this chapter:

- Everyone needs to contribute to a healthy society
- Life skills to interact in the world in healthy ways
- Individuals and communities are inter-dependent
- Skills, infrastructure and principles of operation
- Transformational moments offer opportunities to (re)learn life skills

  - o New parents
  - o School children
  - o Elders

- Different models of local health communities
- Local health communities develop in non-linear ways
- Whole-society participation

Everyone needs to contribute to a healthy society

The theory chapters above (13–19) portray a world of immense complexity. Not only is everything changing in response to everything else, everything is interlinked so there is no end to the work to be done. Carving up the work to make it more manageable simply creates new silos that is the very problem that integrated care is trying to solve.

Rather than hard-wire everything together, strategy needs to help people to *dip in and out of each other's lives, promoting alignment, synchronicity, mutuality, reciprocity and co-adaptation.* But the scale is vast. A healthy society requires all agencies and citizens, not merely health services, to contribute to care and health promotion, and align their efforts with those of others. Furthermore, we need ongoing opportunities to do this because everything is continually changing. When a new system is in place, people settle into the new routine, but that new routine quickly becomes the old routine as new things happen. *A multi-level, whole-society strategy for ongoing co-evolution is needed.*

Also huge is the number of people we need to engage, and the number of people who lack the most basic skills and understanding of facilitating collaboration at scale. Even those who want to develop a more equitable and less selfish society often lack knowledge and experience of how to go about it. *Society needs to help citizens to learn and relearn at every stage of life the skills of being a systems-aware team player.*

Also formidable is the pressure on general practice. Asking more of an already overwhelmed discipline at first sight seems unrealistic. However, the models presented in this book show how to ease the pressure on primary care teams with a systematic approach to *self-care, shared care* and *collaborative health promotion.* Formative and ongoing training of primary care practitioners should prepare them for their part in this.

This chapter proposes a way to spread the load of care and health promotion more broadly throughout society. It proposes annual cycles of inter-organisational learning and change led by different groups and supported by primary care and public health. These aim to nurture local communities for health. It proposes a set of skills that help people to engage in the cycles in productive ways. These same skills help people to interact with others in appreciative, creative and equal ways. These skills should be learned and re-learned at all stages of life by all citizens.

Life skills to interact in the world in healthy ways

Chapter 15 suggests a set of life skills that help people to interact in a complex world in ways that develop trusted relationships and healthy life stories. These same skills are needed by team players and leadership teams for integrated care. The skills are to:

1   **Be alive in the moment:** Appreciate that the world is complex and continually changing, and remain balanced and alert within this turbulence. Dis-eases can challenge this sense of vitality, but can also be used to creatively enhance it. We learn this skill by practising techniques that calm our inner anxieties, listening at a deep level, being grateful for what we have rather than resentful of things we lack, seeing things from different perspectives and seizing opportunities to nudge things in good directions.

2   **Adventure in an uncertain world:** Live life forwards with optimism, appreciate the people we are travelling with, use techniques that help to inquire into complex situations, learn from experience and use all of these to turn bad into good. We learn this skill through different kinds of life experience, leading participatory action research projects, thoughtful planning and networks of trusted relationships.

3   **Be a team player:** Dip in and out of different kinds of project, and adopt different team roles to make timely contributions that make wholes more than the sum of the parts. Build healthy communities and judge people for who they are rather than who they are not. We learn this skill through team-learning, whole-system thinking and by contributing to shared leadership teams, and networks of such teams.

4   **Be a life-long, life-wide learner:** Reflect on experience and change our behaviours accordingly. See whole systems as well as detailed aspects and maintain the coherence of our life stories. We learn this skill by reflecting on experience, and inter-generational learning – learning from and with those who are different from us. We listen more than we speak. We trust more than we distrust. We think at different levels. We see connections between wholes and parts. We make sense of facts within broader stories.

5   **Be resilient:** Bend like a reed in the wind without breaking under pressure and remain centred when things are turbulent – surfing the waves of life. We learn this skill by testing ourselves at increasing levels of difficulty with different kinds of challenge, both at work and at home. We go with the flow in ways that retain a degree of control and direction.

These skills help us to juggle many 'balls' at the same time, and see patterns in complex situations that help us to pick good paths through the mess of life.

The skills help to develop teams and networks of teams that make a difference. They help to identify sets of coordinated actions that achieve different things at the same time – treat diseases, help ourselves, contribute to the efforts of others, and so on. We learn to 'think globally and act locally', to care for the environment, to care for ourselves and for those around us.

It involves deep listening – to what others say and also to what they mean to say yet struggle to put into words. It also involves listening to *ourselves* and asking ourselves if what we say is really what we mean. This helps us to try out new ways of thinking and acting. This is how individuals grow. It is how teams, groups and communities grow.

The skills to take part and lead such processes of learning and change can be learned at any age. Some have better innate skills, but everyone can continually improve.

Individuals and communities are inter-dependent

In the twentieth century there developed an idea that individuals and communities are separate entities. You either believe in individualism or collectivism. Similarly, capitalism and communism became thought of as opposed to each other.

Chapters 15 and 18 challenge these polarities. Individuals naturally interact in the world to develop webs of relationships. This is how we develop our identities. Webs of relationships *are* communities – healthy or not. Individuals and communities do not stand alone. They are inter-linked realities, examined with different lenses.

The inter-dependence of individuals and communities explains why people must have *responsibilities as well as rights*. Everyone needs to be concerned about the welfare of others because this affects their own well-being – it is *enlightened self-interest*. People often do this only for their own 'kind' – their family, discipline, ideology, gender, community. The challenge for policy is to help people to feel a broader sense of responsibility for the world beyond their immediate concerns.

Another unhelpful twentieth-century polarisation is how to go about social control. One says that entirely top-down control is needed, citing people's tendency to be selfish. Another says that entirely bottom-up entrepreneurs are needed, citing Adam Smith's *invisible hand* to explain how markets have self-balancing mechanisms. But each, on its own, causes fragmentation. The first puts people directly into silos; the second leaves the entrepreneurs to do it.

Here, a third way is proposed. A way that enables complex co-adaptations. Annual cycles of collaborative improvement within local health communities allow people from different backgrounds to dip in and out of each other's lives. The intention is not to control each other, but to better understand each other and align their ways of thinking and working. They do this by aligning their calendars and doing small things together. Everyone retains their own centre of gravity, but they also come to realise that with small adjustments they can make their combined impacts more than their individual contributions. And if people don't do what they have agreed, the punitive aspect kicks in.

An infrastructure of facilitation and communication is needed to maintain such cycles. This includes *learning sets* and *leadership courses* that help multidisciplinary leadership teams to learn from each other and influence change across larger areas. Participants in the learning sets and courses learn how to engage large numbers of people in community building by scheduling a series of connected events that incrementally build shared vision and a culture of collaboration. They learn how to evaluate whole-system cohesion and work with strategic partners to support developments.

Participation in the process of building communities helps people to develop skills to interact with others in mutually enhancing ways. This turns individual 'I' into collective 'we'. The same skills need to be re-learned at every stage of life, from childhood to end of life. Primary and secondary schools, universities and postgraduate education should add these skills to their curricula, not merely because it is good for society – it is in their self-interest for their students to be strong as individuals and as community members.

Skills, infrastructure and principles of operation

A central argument emerges from the previous chapters – community-oriented integrated care (COIC) that includes health promotion is desirable, but not easy to achieve. It requires everyone to engage in processes of team and community development that build networks of trusted relationships throughout whole systems of care and within geographic communities. It requires citizens, leaders and policy-makers to want to work for the system as a whole, beyond their self-interest. The following help to achieve this:

Individual skills: Individuals need to learn and relearn skills that enable them to:

- Be alive and balanced in the moment, able to adventure in unfamiliar places, be team players, and be resilient, life-long, life-wide learners
- Conceptualise whole systems and coherent stories, see connections between parts and wholes and make timely contributions to enhance both
- Be able to develop equal relationships and diverse communities

Infrastructure: Sustainability requires infrastructure to build and maintain:

- Mechanisms in all parts of society, beyond health care, to support boundary-spanning learning and change for shared care and health promotion
- Networks of multidisciplinary leadership teams to engage people and organisations in coordinated cycles of inter-organisational, inter-disciplinary learning and change
- Applied research units to develop networks of leadership teams to have a combined effect more than the sum of their individual contributions

Principles of operation: Ongoing whole-system integration requires:

- Policy to support the idea that health is everyone's concern and citizens must care about the health of whole populations, beyond their own self-interest

- Organisations to use principles of organisational learning that include cycles of inter-organisational learning and change and a culture of collaboration
- A curriculum of citizenship that includes life skills for an integrated world, revisited at all stages of life, to help citizens to be systems thinkers who are skilled at collaboration

Transformational moments offer opportunities to (re)learn life skills

Chapter 4 lists large numbers of organisations in addition to health care that need to contribute to collaborative care and health improvements – families, faith groups, local authorities, employers, schools, political parties, and so on. Their relevance is particularly obvious at moments of transformation. Transformational moments are times when individuals or groups are ready to change the way they think about themselves and how they relate to others. They are often precipitated by major life events – bolts from the blue and also predictable ones.

To illustrate the potential of transformational moments to help people to learn these life skills, let us here consider three predictable ones: 1) new parents; 2) school children; and 3) elders.

New parents

A new baby is a wonderful experience for new parents that releases strong emotions to care. Quickly parents discover unfamiliar tasks and experiences, like sleepless nights and different opinions about parenting. They often also find unexpected challenges to their relationships, both with each other and with others. Many make the mistake of taking their partner for granted, or forcing rather than negotiating change, with little insight into the consequences of their actions. Unhealthy patterns of behaviour can easily develop that cause long-term harm.

Building a family with a new child is an opportunity to re-learn citizenship skills, for example *adventuring in an uncertain world*. Parents can find new ways to live life forwards with optimism, appreciating their partners and trying out new things that make people happy and healthy. They can use parenting classes, videos and drop-in centres to be reminded that relationships need to be continually refreshed and doing this enriches them as individuals, as families and as citizens (as well as being good role models for their children).

Parent groups are well placed to lead this, supported by maternity services, health visiting services and general practices.

School children

School is a profound step in a child's life, when they move from dependence to mature independence, equally comfortable with 'I' and 'we'. Whatever the parents think is important for a child to learn, in school hours the teacher is in charge. Poor outcomes come both from leaving education entirely in teachers' hands, and also from leaving it entirely in parents' hands. A partnership between parents and teachers is needed.

Recognising that school is a transformational moment for families helps parents and teachers as well as children to re-learn citizenship skills, for example *being a team player*. Acting on this means making the home a learning environment, working with teachers to enhance the learning of their child, and working with other parents and staff to make the school work well. Schools can support drop-in mornings to discuss a range of health matters. A sequence of community-building events can be overseen by a range of leadership teams – parent–staff liaison, sports, music, outings, art, and so on. Parent council, children council and staff council can meet throughout the year to discuss strategy.

Schools can help children to learn the full range of skills to interact in the world in healthy ways. They can learn from music and sport how to combine harmony and control. They can use group projects to learn to value different perspectives, listen at a deep level, negotiate, co-adapt and adopt different roles in teams. They can interview and shadow people from different backgrounds to see how different contexts produce different challenges. Through outward bound activities that can learn how to adventure in a complex world, and see connections between parts and wholes. They can use role play, debate and creative activities to learn every kind of communication skill.

Schools and parents are well placed to lead this, supported by local authorities and children's services.

Elders

In his final book, Erikson revised his list of eight life transformations to describe a ninth – old age. The things we were once able to do effortlessly are now difficult. Coming to terms with failing faculties and difficulty in doing new things, and at the same time having significant life experience and wisdom can make us depressed and lonely. We have to face up to these challenges by finding new interests and ways to make sense of our lives as whole stories.

This transformational moment affects the individuals concerned, their families, and also the various communities to which they belong. Life skills of *being alive in the moment* and *being a life-long, life-wide learner* help them to make sense of their life stories. Those who support the elderly can help them to 'make the third age the best age' by developing new interests, keeping active and making practical contributions to community life. In addition, they can reminisce, or write their memoirs, or describe their adventures to a grandchild who is doing their school project on citizenship.

Voluntary agencies are well placed to lead this, supported by families and social services.

Different models of local health communities

Chapters 1 and 13 describe models of collaboration between health care and the rest of society to build local health communities within which parents, children, the elderly and everyone else contribute to a healthy society. Quebec's local health networks, Mead's community development agencies, UK's Vanguard sites and others all aim to do this.

The model of *local health community* proposed here is a geographic area of about 50,000, within which partner organisations agree to collaborate for health promotion and shared care. Within this locality, shared leadership teams lead four stakeholder events each year (February, April, July and November). At these, participants review their shared vision, feed-back learning from projects, attend workshops to learn new things, and devise care plans and improvement projects. They are dynamic events where participants move between tables and rooms, guided by their 'two feet'. The overall effect is to refresh relationships as well as get a lot of work done. Inter-organisational collaborative projects are modest and easily achieved, since their main purpose is to achieve synchrony of effort, rather than overly time-consuming new work.

A multidisciplinary shared leadership team meets monthly to keep things happening in between the larger events. It sends a monthly update to three contacts in each partner organisation who are responsible to cascade information. The model includes practice leadership teams, locality leadership teams and system leadership teams that become a network of leadership teams with broad reach. A learning set helps the teams to learn from and with each other about how to lead integrated care and health promotion.

Whatever the model, it is worth involving general practices and public health in some way, because they link with statutory services for individual and population health and care. Many other organisations will also need to be involved depending on the issues of the moment.

Local health communities develop in non-linear ways

Different models of local health community naturally develop in ways that fit well with the local context. Progress is not linear. This is illustrated by the model proposed in this book. Its development happened in ways that were not planned and only with hindsight made sense as a coherent story. In the moment, developments were disjointed, often going backwards. Future direction emerged from unexpected events and opportunities seized upon by those who were around. Only with hindsight were the originating threads discernible.

In 2008, a primary care trust (PCT) in a west London borough (Ealing) wanted to improve collaboration between public health and primary care. The borough had 70 general practices that served a population of about 330,000. Joint planning between public health and primary care directorates led to health-promotion projects, research practices and using the Joint Strategic Needs Assessment (written by Public Health) to plan primary care development.

Between 2009 and 2012, the PCT piloted a local health community. A team facilitated collaboration between 23 general practices in Southall, a geographic area of 65,000 population. They took part in annual cycles of collective reflection and co-ordinated action within which they co-designed system improvements. The four main institutions relating to general practice were invited to take part – mental health, acute care, social care and community care. It was called Southall Initiative for Integrated Care. Leadership came from multidisciplinary teams that spanned the organisations and disciplines of the participants.

Southall Initiative for Integrated Care led to five projects. All were shaped by the 23 general practices in Southall, working in four quadrants, each of about six practices. They were:

1   Implementing a dementia strategy, including early diagnosis and ongoing monitoring of elderly patients with cognitive impairment

2   Developing community links for the support of children and families
3   Implementing the local diabetes strategy, including diabetic clinics in general practice
4   Treating anxiety and depression in black and minority ethnic populations
5   Aligning data from various computer systems to locality boundaries

This experience led to a recognition that an effective local health community needs to be aligned to cultural and geographic boundaries. An area of about 50,000 is a good 'village' size for collaborative activities in a UK city. The PCT acted on this to negotiate with all its GPs to cluster into areas of about this size. Negotiators examined things like bus routes, arterial roads, industrial estates and availability of meeting rooms, to identify natural configurations. Ealing tentatively sketched out seven localities.

Planning for localities to export learning from the Southall Initiative for Integrated Care ended in March 2011 when the PCT closed and the clinical commissioning group (CCG) began, bringing new priorities. However, in July 2011, an entirely different initiative – the North-West London Integrated Care Pilot (ICP) – gave impetus for a next stage. It funded general practices in localities of about 50,000 population to meet as multi-disciplinary groups (MDGs) to develop care plans for patients at risk of hospital admission.

The ICP gave the CCG an opportunity to bring seven localities into being. They were called 'health networks' to signal intention to collaborate for medical matters (rather than local health communities that would be concerned about broader health issues). For each, the CCG appointed two 'MDG chairs' who convened the monthly meetings. A leadership course for the chairs, based on principles of work-based learning, was commissioned by the CCG.

An innovation fund was set up in 2012, overseen by a group that included the MDG chairs. This raised awareness of the need to target health-promotion initiatives at times when people are ready for change (transformational moments). One of the many successful projects, led by Age Concern, was to set up a befriending service for elders, especially because many elderly people were socially isolated. However, the arrangements did not include pilot testing with any particular health network and the opportunity for continued advocacy and development of the initiative was missed. This raised awareness of the need for a collaborative approach when developing initiatives.

From 2012, momentum for integration gathered throughout the UK. General practices in many parts of the UK started to cluster into geographic areas, recognising that this aided collaboration. In 2013 the ICP became renamed as the Whole Systems Integrated Care (WSIC) as one of 14 'pioneers' launched by the coalition government in 2013 to remove barriers to integrated care. In 2014, the nationally negotiated New GP contract required general practices to case manage 2 per cent of their patients most at risk of being admitted to hospital, giving further impetus to multidisciplinary collaboration.

In 2015, the monthly meetings of health networks changed to four times a year, for reasons of funding and time. One of the seven – Central Ealing Health Network – was given permission to pilot the processes of the Southall Initiative for Integrated Care, with the intention of exploring ways to change *health networks* into *local health communities*.

At the same time, in an entirely different west London borough (Brent), a school developed a monthly drop-in meeting to discuss a range of health issues, mainly parenting. Its local health network supported this. One of the many issues raised was sleep problems. By coincidence, a friend of one of the parents made parenting videos about a range of health issues, including sleep problems. Over some months, discussions at school drop-in meetings and parties resulted in these videos being offered free to parents of the (Brent) school and also to patients of the ten general practices in Central Ealing Health Network.

This led to four 2016 collaborations: collaboration with Essential Parent Company, pharmacists, out-of-hours practitioners and mental health practitioners. These paved the way for a set of projects in 2017 that included:

1   **Parenting videos:** This includes free access to patients via the general practice website. Evaluation included downloads by practice, adjusted for practice population. Future developments considered at the time included feedback to the company about improvements of the videos, need for videos for other stages of life, and access to the videos through children's centres and health visitors.

2   **Mental health live manual:** This took advantage of redesign of mental health services in west London. The intended outcome was a manual to help practitioners understand what they can do at different stages of life to improve mental health, as well as understand the new system for mental health care. Future developments considered at the time included writing live manuals for other issues, and rolling programmes for new mothers about positive mental health for the whole family.

3   **Public health live manual:** This includes writing a directory of health promotion initiatives led by public health, to be advertised in the waiting rooms of participating general practices. Future developments considered at the time included a rolling programme of self-help courses (e.g. for elders and carers, for people with long-term conditions, and for new mothers).

4   **Partnership with out-of-hours GP service:** This included identifying things that daytime GPs can do to help out-of-hours GPs to contribute to care plans, and things the out-of-hours GPs can do to enhance daytime practice. Future developments considered at the time included working with GP educators to teach leadership of whole-system improvement.

With hindsight this story makes sense, as though deliberately planned for one stage to build from previous ones. Living life forwards, however, it was not at all straightforward. Planned developments did not happen and other ones did. It was the thoughtful actions of people in different parts of the system that adjusted new initiatives to rehabilitate old ideas.

Projects to improve the positive health of parents, families, children and elders *did* happen in this local health community. But they were not specifically planned. They emerged from discussions between those who were 'at the table'.

A lesson from this case study is – don't be too fixed on a specific model or a specific route. Oscillate between the long-term vision and whatever steps are realistic at any moment. And keep going, with optimism.

Whole-society participation

One question is where the leadership will come from to develop local health communities and cycles of inter-organisational learning and change for whole-society health?

General practice and public health do not have the capacity to lead all of this. Nor should they. The geographic nature of local health communities provides opportunities for others to lead parallel initiatives that can be linked at strategic times. Schools, faith groups, voluntary groups and others have their own reasons to lead cycles of collaborative learning and coordinated change. They could develop a loose coalition of partner agencies to inform each other of their locality-based cycles. *Whoever can should lead the development of local health communities, supported by whichever partner agencies want to engage.*

They need infrastructure to support their work. Data, training, advocacy and places to meet are important, and sometimes funding for participation. Shared leadership teams of different kinds need to be systematically developed, with routine ways to pass their roles onto their successors. Applied research units need to develop leadership teams, help them to learn from and with each other, and build a network of facilitative leaders for cultural change. The effect of real-time strategic change and organisational learning needs to be evaluated. *Politicians, universities, commissioning groups and funding bodies could lead this.*

Students of all ages need to develop the skills to participate in collaborative learning and coordinated change for a healthy society. *Educational establishments could lead this.*

There is an international need to share insights into humane, low-conflict ways to integrate human efforts for health and care. The ability of organisational learning principles to support this needs to be considered seriously and models evaluated. Issues like global warming, non-renewable resources, refugees and ethnic conflicts are all health issues that might be helped by this kind of thinking. An international network of collaborating sites needs to enable discussions about effective models.

In the UK we need to explore ways for general practices and public health to work with local authorities, schools, faith groups, voluntary groups, politicians, business and others to develop local health communities, and with this to stimulate vibrant, mature debate at local levels about creating a healthy society. This is a form of participatory democracy.

We need to pilot connected cycles of collaborative learning and coordinated change led by different organisations. Some may develop in parallel, with token overlap; others may have strategic linkage, perhaps with stakeholder events that last several days, or use real-time strategic change (Chapter 10) to continue interaction over months and years.

Whatever models may emerge, they will always need to combine a breadth of insight and a philosophy of co-evolution. Neither top-down protocols nor bottom-up entrepreneurs are enough. *Community-oriented integrated care* needs predicable processes of engagement and also ways to creatively interact. Leadership teams must have elbow room to shape what happens and achieve useful things – things that keep people thinking outwards as well as inwards, and trying out new things. We need to weave together our personal insights, top-down policy, objective data and bottom-up energy.

We will need to seize opportunities of the moment. We will need to be bold.

Appendix
Skills to lead community-oriented integrated care

Complete the questionnaire with your project in mind

The best way to approach this questionnaire is with a project in mind that you intend to lead. This will help you to distinguish between the things you *need* to learn for practical reasons, and the things you *want* to learn for more general interest.

For every learning objective identify how confident you feel at present, and how important it is for you to learn *within one year*. In the comment section, indicate things you would like to put on your five-year 'wish list' (and anything else you want; this is not a test, you are writing for yourself).

At the end, go back and choose *two* objectives from each of the four sections that you want to commit to learn within one year. Add these to your learning plan at the end. Consider especially those that you have scored 'unconfident' and 'very important' – these are likely to be things you don't want to learn, but need to.

This will give you eight priority learning objectives for the year and many more on your 'wish-list'. Keep your answers safe because you will want to revisit them in future years to add and remove learning objectives from your wish list (you will be surprised how many you achieve along the way without specifically planning to).

The best way to learn your chosen objectives is through your project(s). It helps to stand back and reflect immediately after having tried something out (or at least within two days), listing things that went well and things you would do differently next time (in that order – positive first). Ideally, do this with people who were involved, and who will give you trustworthy feedback. It is also useful to reflect with those who are leading similar projects (e.g. on a leadership course).

Some definitions

Integrated care means care that is coordinated across organisational and disciplinary boundaries. Practitioners on all sides of all the boundaries being crossed enjoy good relationships that enable creative team-working and synchronised ongoing improvements. Each organisation creates policy that enables good communication and collaborative improvements with practitioners on the ground.

Community-oriented integrated care means integrated care and health promotion that is oriented towards local communities. Geographic areas of 30–50,000 populations are a good size for organisations such as general practices, schools, businesses and voluntary groups to work together for shared care.

Health promotion means everything to do with improving health for individuals, networks and communities. It means more than care of people with illnesses. It includes skills to be alive in the moment and to seize opportunities to nudge things in good directions. It includes developing environments that encourage healthy behaviour – make healthy choices easy choices. It includes developing healthy social networks, from which comes resilience and well-being.

Transformational leadership means changing whole systems as well as its parts. Transformational leaders are sense-makers – they help people to appreciate why integration matters and how to achieve it. They model collaborative behaviour and use participatory approaches to learning and change. They persuade people to collaborate and make it easy for them to do so. They shape shared projects for whole-system improvement. They create and maintain infrastructure to support continuous quality improvements. They apply transformational principles in their own lives.

Skills to lead COIC are described under five broad learning aims

1 Concepts for community-oriented integrated care (COIC)

    1.1 Trends in health care
    1.2 Three aspects of reality
    1.3 Creative interactions between different perspectives
    1.4 How organisations, networks and systems learn and change

2 Evaluating COIC

    2.1 Bringing connections into view
    2.2 Assess team skills
    2.3 Research methods for transformational change
    2.4 Identify your own needs for personal transformation

3 Facilitating learning spaces

    3.1 Facilitate learning in groups
    3.2 Facilitate learning in a network
    3.3 Facilitate a large group event
    3.4 Bring dynamic interactions into view

4 Orchestrating whole-system learning and change

    4.1 Lead system-transforming projects
    4.2 Build infrastructure that facilitates ongoing learning and change
    4.3 Manage coordinated sets of projects
    4.4 Feed-back useful data at appropriate times

5 Skills for personal balance

    5.1 Interact with others in ways that develop healthy stories
    5.2 Retain inner peace
    5.3 Maintain a network of personal and political support
    5.4 Maintain systems to manage information

1 Concepts for community-oriented integrated care (COIC)

Leaders need to be able to explain why community-oriented integrated care is important and its history. They need to explain its science – approaches to research and development that illuminate processes of multiple human interaction from which emerge trusted relationships, meaning and innovation. They need to relate these concepts to health as perceived by individuals in different contexts. This science is poorly understood. Western societies have strong beliefs in a fragmenting approach to knowledge generation and an isolating understanding of identity construction – *positivism* and *individualism*. Relationships, culture and integrated care are invisible to these ways of thinking, except as mechanical transactions and contracts. Other theories are needed to illuminate dynamic co-adaptation, emergence and transformation.

1.1 Trends in health care

1.1.1 Comprehensive primary health care

This is a term agreed at the 1978 conference at Alma Ata to describe holistic health care, of which medical care is a part.

Unconfident   Confident
1 [ ]   2 [ ]   3 [ ]   4 [ ]

Not important in the next year   Very important in the next year
1 [ ]   2 [ ]   3 [ ]   4 [ ]

Comment:

1.1.2 Origins of general practice before the NHS: 1858–1948

Unconfident   Confident
1 [ ]   2 [ ]   3 [ ]   4 [ ]

Not important in the next year   Very important in the next year
1 [ ]   2 [ ]   3 [ ]   4 [ ]

Comment:

1.1.3 From general practitioner to multidisciplinary community-oriented primary care: 1948–1990

Unconfident   Confident
1 [ ]   2 [ ]   3 [ ]   4 [ ]

Not important in the next year   Very important in the next year
1 [ ]   2 [ ]   3 [ ]   4 [ ]

Comment:

1.1.4 From community-oriented primary care to COIC: 1990–

Unconfident   Confident
1 [ ]   2 [ ]   3 [ ]   4 [ ]

Not important in the next year   Very important in the next year
1 [ ]   2 [ ]   3 [ ]   4 [ ]

Comment:

1.1.5 What generalists do that is different from specialists

Unconfident   Confident
1 [ ]   2 [ ]   3 [ ]   4 [ ]

Not important in the next year   Very important in the next year
1 [ ]   2 [ ]   3 [ ]   4 [ ]

Comment:

1.1.6 Models of primary care organisation

Unconfident   Confident
1 [ ]   2 [ ]   3 [ ]   4 [ ]

Not important in the next year   Very important in the next year
1 [ ]   2 [ ]   3 [ ]   4 [ ]

Comment:

1.1.7 Contemporary health-care policy

Unconfident   Confident
1 [ ]   2 [ ]   3 [ ]   4 [ ]

Not important in the next year   Very important in the next year
1 [ ]   2 [ ]   3 [ ]   4 [ ]

Comment:

1.1.8 What other learning objectives do you have in this topic?

1.2 Three aspects of reality

1.2.1 Positivism, critical theory and constructivism illuminate different aspects of truth

Positivism imagines reality to be made up of discrete particles; truth is seen from simple observation. *Critical theory* imagines that what you see at first sight is interconnected with many other invisible factors; getting at the truth means getting behind the immediately obvious to see hidden connections. *Constructivism* imagines that reality is constantly evolving as multiple interactions adapt to each other; truth is coherence between multiple factors. Each of these *paradigms* requires a different approach to methods and validation. Often all three are valuable.

Unconfident   Confident
1 [ ]   2 [ ]   3 [ ]   4 [ ]

Not important in the next year   Very important in the next year
1 [ ]   2 [ ]   3 [ ]   4 [ ]

Comment:

1.2.2 Predictive, emergent and transformational change

Predictive change means simple cause-and-effect (e.g. a billiard ball hits another). Emergent change means interaction between intimately related things to co-evolve (e.g. a sea-shore). Transformational change means change of a whole system to create something new (e.g. a caterpillar transforms into a butterfly). Emergent change can be an *incremental transformation* when it contributes to change of a whole system.

Unconfident   Confident
1 [ ]   2 [ ]   3 [ ]   4 [ ]

Not important in the next year   Very important in the next year
1 [ ]   2 [ ]   3 [ ]   4 [ ]

Comment:

1.2.3 Hard, soft and whole systems

Referring a diabetic to a specialist uses a 'hard' system idea – like a heart pump the flow is in a predictable direction. In *shared care*, multiple attendants exchange views, using a 'soft system' idea – like multiple movements across a cell membrane. The whole diabetes strategy (like a whole human body) is a whole system in which many different hard and soft systems work in synchrony as a complex integrated system.

Unconfident   Confident
1 [ ]   2 [ ]   3 [ ]   4 [ ]

Not important in the next year   Very important in the next year
1 [ ]   2 [ ]   3 [ ]   4 [ ]

Comment:

1.2.4 Vertical, horizontal and whole-system integration

Vertical integration describes the care pathways that help patients move from the local, generalist environment to specialist care. Horizontal integration describes team-building between disciplines from different care pathways and within local health communities. All contribute to whole system integration

Unconfident   Confident
1 [ ]   2 [ ]   3 [ ]   4 [ ]

Not important in the next year   Very important in the next year
1 [ ]   2 [ ]   3 [ ]   4 [ ]

Comment:

1.2.5 What other learning objectives do you have in this topic?

1.3 Creative interactions between different perspectives

Different perspectives can make sense as a whole through conversations (dialectic) that result in shared stories. Triangulation of data and crystallisation of meaning help to do this.

1.3.1 Different research approaches are different lenses that see different things

Unconfident   Confident
1 [ ]   2 [ ]   3 [ ]   4 [ ]

Not important in next two years   Very important in the next year
1 [ ]   2 [ ]   3 [ ]   4 [ ]

Comment:

1.3.2 Human interaction builds shared stories by moving between parent, adult and child ego states

Unconfident   Confident
1 [ ]   2 [ ]   3 [ ]   4 [ ]

Not important in next two years   Very important in the next year
1 [ ]   2 [ ]   3 [ ]   4 [ ]

Comment:

1.3.3 Narrative unity determines health, meaning, motivation and identity

Health is a holistic concept, in which all aspects of a life story make sense to each other as a positive 'narrative unity'. Diseases get in the way of that healthy coherence, but they are not health itself. In pursuit of an integrated sense of self (identity) we pursue narrative unity because it is meaningful to us; we are motivated by maintaining and extending that sense of coherence.

Unconfident			Confident
1 [ ]	2 [ ]	3 [ ]	4 [ ]

Not important in the next year			Very important in the next year
1 [ ]	2 [ ]	3 [ ]	4 [ ]

Comment:

1.3.4 What other learning objectives do you have in this topic?

1.4 How organisations, systems and communities learn and change

Learning is a cyclical process that reflects practical experience against facts and theories and from this testing out new ways to do things. Neither theory nor experience is enough on its own. Like individuals, organisations, communities and systems learn through such cycles. The cycles also build teams and an organisational culture of learning and collaboration.

1.4.1 Senge's five disciplines

Unconfident			*Confident*
1 [ ]	2 [ ]	3 [ ]	4 [ ]

Not important in the next year			Very important in the next year
1 [ ]	2 [ ]	3 [ ]	4 [ ]

Comment:

1.4.2 Kolb's learning cycle

Unconfident			*Confident*
1 [ ]	2 [ ]	3 [ ]	4 [ ]

Not important in the next year			Very important in the next year
1 [ ]	2 [ ]	3 [ ]	4 [ ]

Comment:

1.4.3 Argyris and Schon's *single-loop, double-loop and deutero-learning in* learning organisations

'Single-loop learning' means the clarification of facts; 'double-loop learning' surfaces hidden and interconnected factors; deutero-learning is the process of innovation through interaction of ideas (also called 'learning-how-to-learn').

Unconfident   Confident
1 [ ]   2 [ ]   3 [ ]   4 [ ]

Not important in the next year   Very important in the next year
1 [ ]   2 [ ]   3 [ ]   4 [ ]

Comment:

1.4.4 Learning organisations, learning networks, learning communities

A general practice or other primary care organisation can work with the principles of organisational learning (or 'become a learning organisation'). Learning networks reach outside of the organisation to connect people with a shared interest; learning communities have a broad range of interests.

Unconfident   Confident
1 [ ]   2 [ ]   3 [ ]   4 [ ]

Not important in the next year   Very important in the next year
1 [ ]   2 [ ]   3 [ ]   4 [ ]

Comment:

1.4.5 What other learning objectives do you have in this topic?

2 Evaluating COIC

Different approaches to evaluation shine different lights on a situation that is actually more complex than any light can reveal on its own.

2.1 Bringing connections into view

2.1.1 Draw a diagram of the whole system concerned – a system map

Using a flip chart or software such as Scenario Generator, draw the connections within a whole system. This allows subsequent analysis of strengths, weaknesses and forces for change

Unconfident   Confident
1 [ ]   2 [ ]   3 [ ]   4 [ ]

Not important in the next year   Very important in the next year
1 [ ]   2 [ ]   3 [ ]   4 [ ]

Comment:

2.1.2 Lead a brainstorm, 'rainbow', nominal group and evaluation matrix

To make sense of multiple perspectives, a range of hopes and concerns need to be surfaced, categorised, then used to stimulate and evaluate progress. A brainstorm surfaces participants' ideas. Rainbow technique helps participants to categorise them. Nominal grouping and evaluation matrices provides categories for participants to work with

Unconfident   Confident
1 [ ]   2 [ ]   3 [ ]   4 [ ]

Not important in the next year   Very important in the next year
1 [ ]   2 [ ]   3 [ ]   4 [ ]

Comment:

2.1.3 Construct a force-field analysis

This analyses forces for and against change.

Unconfident   Confident
1 [ ]   2 [ ]   3 [ ]   4 [ ]

Not important in the next year   Very important in the next year
1 [ ]   2 [ ]   3 [ ]   4 [ ]

Comment:

2.1.4 Draw a complex power diagram

This analyses multiple interacting forces in different parts of the system.

Unconfident   Confident
1 [ ]   2 [ ]   3 [ ]   4 [ ]

Not important in the next year   Very important in the next year
1 [ ]   2 [ ]   3 [ ]   4 [ ]

Comment:

2.1.5 What other learning objectives do you have in this topic?

2.2 Assess team skills

When interviewing for new people to join a team, it helps to focus on how they will fit in. This can be done by formal testing and also by observing interaction. This process also helps established teams to review their teamworking perhaps with an internal facilitator or an external consultant. Teams can score themselves and work together to explore new ways of working informed by the exercises.

2.2.1 Assess roles in teams

Techniques such as Myers Briggs, Belbin, and Honey and Mumford provide useful insights into how a team could improve its operating.

Unconfident			Confident
1 [ ]	2 [ ]	3 [ ]	4 [ ]

Not important in the next year			Very important in the next year
1 [ ]	2 [ ]	3 [ ]	4 [ ]

Comment:

2.2.2 Interview for team players

This combines a) observation of performance in group learning situation, b) presentations and c) open questions, usually as part of a job interview.

Unconfident			Confident
1 [ ]	2 [ ]	3 [ ]	4 [ ]

Not important in the next year			Very important in the next year
1 [ ]	2 [ ]	3 [ ]	4 [ ]

Comment:

2.2.3 Devise in-tray tests

This is a set of real-life tests, usually as part of a job interview.

Unconfident			Confident
1 [ ]	2 [ ]	3 [ ]	4 [ ]

Not important in the next year			Very important in the next year
1 [ ]	2 [ ]	3 [ ]	4 [ ]

Comment:

2.2.4 Goldfish bowl

This comprises real-life team observations of team interactions.

Unconfident			Confident
1 [ ]	2 [ ]	3 [ ]	4 [ ]

Not important in the next year			Very important in the next year
1 [ ]	2 [ ]	3 [ ]	4 [ ]

Comment:

2.2.5 What other learning objectives do you have in this topic?

2.3 Research methods for transformational change

2.3.1 Undertake a rapid appraisal

Unconfident			Confident
1 [ ]	2 [ ]	3 [ ]	4 [ ]

Not important in the next year			Very important in the next year
1 [ ]	2 [ ]	3 [ ]	4 [ ]

Comment:

2.3.2 Lead a participatory action research project

Unconfident			Confident
1 [ ]	2 [ ]	3 [ ]	4 [ ]

Not important in the next year			Very important in the next year
1 [ ]	2 [ ]	3 [ ]	4 [ ]

Comment:

2.3.3 Know the strengths and weaknesses of different research methods

Unconfident			Confident
1 [ ]	2 [ ]	3 [ ]	4 [ ]

Not important in the next year			Very important in the next year
1 [ ]	2 [ ]	3 [ ]	4 [ ]

Comment:

2.3.4 Evaluate projects using quantitative, qualitative and participatory insights

Unconfident			Confident
1 [ ]	2 [ ]	3 [ ]	4 [ ]

Not important in the next year			Very important in the next year
1 [ ]	2 [ ]	3 [ ]	4 [ ]

Comment:

2.3.5 Devise a case study of COIC

Unconfident   Confident
1 [ ]   2 [ ]   3 [ ]   4 [ ]

Not important in the next year   Very important in the next year
1 [ ]   2 [ ]   3 [ ]   4 [ ]

Comment:

2.3.6 What other learning objectives do you have in this topic?

2.4 Identifying your own needs for personal transformation

Personal transformation means changing the way you think about yourself and your interaction with others. It involves rewriting your life script in a way that is healthier, uses a better set of mental models and is better able to see yourself as others see you. Personal transformation can be confusing and painful – an 'existential crisis' – as though the old self has to die and a new self reborn. Worth doing this within a therapeutic relationship of some kind.

2.4.1 Draw a personal life journey

This helps to review your own life story which might reveal your hidden motivations and mental models that are holding you back.

Unconfident   Confident
1 [ ]   2 [ ]   3 [ ]   4 [ ]

Not important in the next year   Very important in the next year
1 [ ]   2 [ ]   3 [ ]   4 [ ]

Comment:

2.4.2 Deal with projection

It is common for people to project their ways of thinking and feeling onto others, often attributing to others traits that are more truthfully their own. Can you deal with this well? Do you project in this way?

Unconfident   Confident
1 [ ]   2 [ ]   3 [ ]   4 [ ]

Not important in the next year   Very important in the next year
1 [ ]   2 [ ]   3 [ ]   4 [ ]

Comment:

2.4.3 Reflect on your daily experiences, identify aspects of the environment that support good practice, pilot improvements and evaluate them

Unconfident			Confident
1 [ ]	2 [ ]	3 [ ]	4 [ ]

Not important in the next year			Very important in the next year
1 [ ]	2 [ ]	3 [ ]	4 [ ]

Comment:

2.4.4 Anticipate your own future support needs and make them happen

Unconfident			Confident
1 [ ]	2 [ ]	3 [ ]	4 [ ]

Not important in the next year			Very important in the next year
1 [ ]	2 [ ]	3 [ ]	4 [ ]

Comment:

2.4.5 What other learning objectives do you have in this topic?

3 Facilitating learning spaces

Leaders must be able to help people to learn from and with each other in small groups, large groups and in transformational projects. Often bespoke events need to be designed but they can be usefully informed by established models. For example, Future Search explores shared vision and Open Space facilitates self-organisation. Real-Time Strategic Change can be used to allow real-life teams to interact at one event, or over time within a transformational project.

3.1 Facilitate learning in groups

3.1.1 Chair and facilitate a meeting, and know the difference between the two styles

Unconfident			Confident
1 [ ]	2 [ ]	3 [ ]	4 [ ]

Not important in the next year			Very important in the next year
1 [ ]	2 [ ]	3 [ ]	4 [ ]

Comment:

3.1.2 Prepare a check-list for a meeting – a list of easy-to-forget things

Unconfident   Confident
1 [ ]   2 [ ]   3 [ ]   4 [ ]

Not important in the next year   Very important in the next year
1 [ ]   2 [ ]   3 [ ]   4 [ ]

Comment:

3.1.3 Use backwards mapping to devise learning objectives

Unconfident   Confident
1 [ ]   2 [ ]   3 [ ]   4 [ ]

Not important in the next year   Very important in the next year
1 [ ]   2 [ ]   3 [ ]   4 [ ]

Comment:

3.1.4 Centre a learning space – story, energisers, ground rules, evaluation

Unconfident   Confident
1 [ ]   2 [ ]   3 [ ]   4 [ ]

Not important in the next year   Very important in the next year
1 [ ]   2 [ ]   3 [ ]   4 [ ]

Comment:

3.1.5 Facilitate a focus group

Unconfident   Confident
1 [ ]   2 [ ]   3 [ ]   4 [ ]

Not important in the next year   Very important in the next year
1 [ ]   2 [ ]   3 [ ]   4 [ ]

Comment:

3.1.6 What other learning objectives do you have in this topic?

3.2 Facilitate learning in a network

3.2.1 Lead a regular interactive bulletin

Unconfident   Confident
1 [ ]   2 [ ]   3 [ ]   4 [ ]

Not important in the next year   Very important in the next year
1 [ ]   2 [ ]   3 [ ]   4 [ ]

Comment:

3.2.2 Lead discussions through a social networking site

Unconfident   Confident
1 [ ]   2 [ ]   3 [ ]   4 [ ]

Not important in the next year   Very important in the next year
1 [ ]   2 [ ]   3 [ ]   4 [ ]

Comment:

3.2.3 Moderate a web-based discussion

Unconfident   Confident
1 [ ]   2 [ ]   3 [ ]   4 [ ]

Not important in the next year   Very important in the next year
1 [ ]   2 [ ]   3 [ ]   4 [ ]

Comment:

3.2.4 Evaluate learning in groups

Unconfident   Confident
1 [ ]   2 [ ]   3 [ ]   4 [ ]

Not important in the next year   Very important in the next year
1 [ ]   2 [ ]   3 [ ]   4 [ ]

Comment:

3.2.5 Embed cycles of reflection and inquiry within an organisation or community

Unconfident   Confident
1 [ ]   2 [ ]   3 [ ]   4 [ ]

Not important in the next year   Very important in the next year
1 [ ]   2 [ ]   3 [ ]   4 [ ]

Comment:

3.2.6 What other learning objectives do you have in this topic?

3.3 Facilitate a large group event

3.3.1 Facilitate a large group event – Open Space, Vision Workshop, Future Search

Unconfident   Confident
1 [ ]   2 [ ]   3 [ ]   4 [ ]

Not important in the next year   Very important in the next year
1 [ ]   2 [ ]   3 [ ]   4 [ ]

Comment:

3.3.2 Devise your own stakeholder conference

Unconfident			Confident
1 [ ]	2 [ ]	3 [ ]	4 [ ]

Not important in the next year			Very important in the next year
1 [ ]	2 [ ]	3 [ ]	4 [ ]

Comment:

3.3.3 Small-group–large-group iterations

This is connecting small-group reflections with whole-group consensus within a conference.

Unconfident			Confident
1 [ ]	2 [ ]	3 [ ]	4 [ ]

Not important in the next year			Very important in the next year
1 [ ]	2 [ ]	3 [ ]	4 [ ]

Comment:

3.3.4 Facilitate Real-Time Strategic Change in your case study

Unconfident			Confident
1 [ ]	2 [ ]	3 [ ]	4 [ ]

Not important in the next year			Very important in the next year
1 [ ]	2 [ ]	3 [ ]	4 [ ]

Comment:

3.3.5 What other learning objectives do you have in this topic?

3.4 Bring dynamic interactions into view

3.4.1 Lead a role-play, scenario or simulation

Unconfident			Confident
1 [ ]	2 [ ]	3 [ ]	4 [ ]

Not important in the next year			Very important in the next year
1 [ ]	2 [ ]	3 [ ]	4 [ ]

Comment:

3.4.2 Facilitate a goldfish bowl

Unconfident   Confident
1 [ ]   2 [ ]   3 [ ]   4 [ ]

Not important in the next year   Very important in the next year
1 [ ]   2 [ ]   3 [ ]   4 [ ]

Comment:

3.4.3 Construct a digital story and help others to do the same

Tell a story in a few minutes using images, speech and other media.

Unconfident   Confident
1 [ ]   2 [ ]   3 [ ]   4 [ ]

Not important in the next year   Very important in the next year
1 [ ]   2 [ ]   3 [ ]   4 [ ]

Comment:

3.4.4 Draw a system diagram

This helps people to visualise a whole system.

Unconfident   Confident
1 [ ]   2 [ ]   3 [ ]   4 [ ]

Not important in the next year   Very important in the next year
1 [ ]   2 [ ]   3 [ ]   4 [ ]

Comment:

3.4.5 Use backward mapping to develop organisational strategy

Work out what is needed at the most peripheral point and devise support for this to be achieved.

Unconfident   Confident
1 [ ]   2 [ ]   3 [ ]   4 [ ]

Not important in the next year   Very important in the next year
1 [ ]   2 [ ]   3 [ ]   4 [ ]

Comment:

3.4.6 What other learning objectives do you have in this topic?

4 Orchestrating whole-system learning and change

Whole-system transformation requires synchronous changes in many disciplines and organisations. Engaging people from all parts of a system in cycles of learning and change can incrementally achieve transformation. Projects can be led by one organisation (e.g. a diabetic clinic within a general practice), a network (e.g. placing students in a local health community), or a whole system (e.g. elderly care throughout a borough).

The system to be transformed may not be clear at the outset, and the final shape may also be initially unclear. Indeed, change in response to inquiry and learning is a marker of quality and an essential aspect of transformation. To get started a leadership team needs to:

a) Identify relevant people (stakeholders) from all parts of the system and find ways to repeatedly engage them, working with their concerns and hopes.
b) Facilitate a workshop(s) at which stakeholders listen to each other's perspectives, develop shared vision and agree mechanisms to allow the conversation to continue longer term.
c) Form an oversight team that includes the disciplines and organisations that need to contribute to change, and a shared leadership team to lead the next stage. Schedule a sequence of meetings to review progress.
d) Draw a diagram of how the people in a 'whole system' presently connect, and another to show how they *should* re-connect in the envisioned new system. Identify what data need to be gathered to understand what is happening at each part of the system.

The team then leads a rapid appraisal (interviews, observations and literature) to quickly form a view about the strengths and weaknesses of the system as it presently is, and establish the appetite for change. Through three (or more) stakeholder workshops, participants:

a) Redraw the future system map to better reflect the improvements they wish to make
b) Pilot coordinated changes
c) Gather data about what happens in all parts of the system
d) Train everyone how to use the system
e) Provide guidance on maintaining the system in an accessible place (e.g. a website)

At least three cycles of coordinated improvements are needed. Plan for these at the outset.

Cycles of coordinated inter-organisational improvements should continue forever, as the routine way to operate. This allows projects to emerge from an annual calendar of events that are scheduled long in advance, allowing people to engage and disengage at the most appropriate times.

4.1 Lead system-transforming projects

To lead change throughout a system, you have to identify what the system is, who are its stakeholders and who has authority to lead change within it. Then you have to facilitate dialogue between the stakeholders that gets them to agree the rationale for change, a vision for change and steps towards the vision. Through a series of (at least three) cycles of collective reflection and coordinated action (termed participatory action research) they try out new ways of working, gather data about improvements and act on what they have learned.

4.1.1 Enter and exit a system to lead three cycles of participatory action research

Unconfident   Confident
1 [ ]   2 [ ]   3 [ ]   4 [ ]

Not important in the next year   Very important in the next year
1 [ ]   2 [ ]   3 [ ]   4 [ ]

Comment:

4.1.2 Facilitate conversations between stakeholders through interactive bulletins, social networking websites or similar

Unconfident   Confident
1 [ ]   2 [ ]   3 [ ]   4 [ ]

Not important in the next year   Very important in the next year
1 [ ]   2 [ ]   3 [ ]   4 [ ]

Comment:

4.1.3 Facilitate a series of meetings with constituents to develop a project

Unconfident   Confident
1 [ ]   2 [ ]   3 [ ]   4 [ ]

Not important in the next year   Very important in the next year
1 [ ]   2 [ ]   3 [ ]   4 [ ]

Comment:

4.1.4 Facilitate a sequence of stakeholder conferences to coordinate system inter-organisational learning and change

Unconfident   Confident
1 [ ]   2 [ ]   3 [ ]   4 [ ]

Not important in the next year   Very important in the next year
1 [ ]   2 [ ]   3 [ ]   4 [ ]

Comment:

4.1.5 Use an appropriate range of techniques to analyse and overcome obstacles to success of a set of projects (e.g. force-field analysis or complex power diagram)

Unconfident   Confident
1 [ ]   2 [ ]   3 [ ]   4 [ ]

Not important in the next year   Very important in the next year
1 [ ]   2 [ ]   3 [ ]   4 [ ]

Comment:

4.1.6 What other learning objectives do you have in this topic?

4.2 Build infrastructure that facilitates ongoing learning and change

Infrastructure is a forever thing. For integrated care to work, people need an ongoing facility for creative interaction and team-building across organisational boundaries and throughout whole systems of care. They need to be able to access a range of information when they need it.

4.2.1 Build health networks and local health communities

This is best done in a locality of 30–50,000 population – small enough to feel a sense of belonging and large enough to have political influence.

Unconfident   Confident
1 [ ]   2 [ ]   3 [ ]   4 [ ]

Not important in the next year   Very important in the next year
1 [ ]   2 [ ]   3 [ ]   4 [ ]

Comment:

4.2.2 Create an applied research function

This should help practitioners and managers to collaborate to lead ongoing service improvements focused on localities.

Unconfident   Confident
1 [ ]   2 [ ]   3 [ ]   4 [ ]

Not important in the next year   Very important in the next year
1 [ ]   2 [ ]   3 [ ]   4 [ ]

Comment:

4.2.3 Design connected learning spaces

This allows learning in one part of the system to be made useful in other parts.

Unconfident   Confident
1 [ ]   2 [ ]   3 [ ]   4 [ ]

Not important in the next year   Very important in the next year
1 [ ]   2 [ ]   3 [ ]   4 [ ]

Comment:

4.2.4 Create networks of high-performing, deeply embedded, teams

Unconfident   Confident
1 [ ]   2 [ ]   3 [ ]   4 [ ]

Not important in the next year   Very important in the next year
1 [ ]   2 [ ]   3 [ ]   4 [ ]

Comment:

4.2.5 Build mechanisms for in-the-moment decision support

Unconfident   Confident
1 [ ]   2 [ ]   3 [ ]   4 [ ]

Not important in the next year   Very important in the next year
1 [ ]   2 [ ]   3 [ ]   4 [ ]

Comment:

4.2.6 What other learning objectives do you have in this topic?

4.3 Manage coordinated sets of projects

'Silo', 'linear' approaches to research and development do one project at a time, each building on insights from the previous one. When aiming for transformational change this is not enough. Cycles of learning and change need to enable multiple synchronous changes in different parts of a system, then review the overall effect by stakeholders with quite different perspectives, from which they shape a suite of next-stage projects for their next stage of co-evolution.

4.3.1 Monitor sets of coordinated projects, including timelines, staff recruitment, review dates, inter-project learning and finances

Unconfident   Confident
1 [ ]   2 [ ]   3 [ ]   4 [ ]

Not important in the next year   Very important in the next year
1 [ ]   2 [ ]   3 [ ]   4 [ ]

Comment:

4.3.2 Complete a sequence of project tasks on time

Unconfident   Confident
1 [ ]   2 [ ]   3 [ ]   4 [ ]

Not important in the next year   Very important in the next year
1 [ ]   2 [ ]   3 [ ]   4 [ ]

Comment:

4.3.3 Write up a completed project for publication

This can be for local eyes only.

Unconfident   Confident
1 [ ]   2 [ ]   3 [ ]   4 [ ]

Not important in the next year   Very important in the next year
1 [ ]   2 [ ]   3 [ ]   4 [ ]

Comment:

4.3.4 Appraise and supervise others to help them to succeed

Unconfident   Confident
1 [ ]   2 [ ]   3 [ ]   4 [ ]

Not important in the next year   Very important in the next year
1 [ ]   2 [ ]   3 [ ]   4 [ ]

Comment:

4.3.5 Evaluate outcomes from projects, using a full range of research methods, including quantitative, qualitative and participatory insights

Unconfident   Confident
1 [ ]   2 [ ]   3 [ ]   4 [ ]

Not important in the next year   Very important in the next year
1 [ ]   2 [ ]   3 [ ]   4 [ ]

Comment:

4.3.6 What other learning objectives do you have in this topic?

4.4 Feed-back useful data at appropriate times

Feedback of information for learning is a key feature of a learning organisation. When facilitating multiple synchronous changes in transformational projects you have to be able to see the 'woods and the trees'. This is helped by setting up information systems that provide you with reliable, useful information at times when you need it.

4.4.1 Devise an annual timeline that anticipates what data is needed, and when, for different purposes

Unconfident   Confident
1 [ ]   2 [ ]   3 [ ]   4 [ ]

Not important in the next year   Very important in the next year
1 [ ]   2 [ ]   3 [ ]   4 [ ]

Comment:

4.4.2 Design multi-purpose databases

This should systematically provide reports from different kinds of data from different parts of the system.

Unconfident   Confident
1 [ ]   2 [ ]   3 [ ]   4 [ ]

Not important in the next year   Very important in the next year
1 [ ]   2 [ ]   3 [ ]   4 [ ]

Comment:

4.4.3 Draw a power diagram to analyse who influences who

Unconfident   Confident
1 [ ]   2 [ ]   3 [ ]   4 [ ]

Not important in the next year   Very important in the next year
1 [ ]   2 [ ]   3 [ ]   4 [ ]

Comment:

4.4.4 Use routinely gathered data to stimulate learning and change in case studies

Unconfident   Confident
1 [ ]   2 [ ]   3 [ ]   4 [ ]

Not important in the next year   Very important in the next year
1 [ ]   2 [ ]   3 [ ]   4 [ ]

Comment:

4.4.5 What other learning objectives do you have in this topic?

5 Skills for personal balance

Leaders of community-oriented integrated care naturally encounter many different opinions. Misunderstandings are common. You can easily become overwhelmed by the scale of operation and the number of demands, as well as the hostility and blame that can accompany those things. To thrive and to continue to be useful to others you have to be able to bend like a reed in the wind when under pressure.

To do this you need inner balance that come from a sense of your own coherent life story, coupled with techniques that help to get inner doubts into perspective. You need to be open and listening to others even when they are distracted by other concerns, using high-level communication skills that are high on impact and low on time. You need to be skilled at distinguishing between things you can control and things you can't, and taking advantage of unexpected events to turn bad into good.

5.1 Interact with others in ways that develop healthy stories

5.1.1 Communicate well with different kinds of people using different media

Unconfident   Confident
1 [ ]   2 [ ]   3 [ ]   4 [ ]

Not important in the next year   Very important in the next year
1 [ ]   2 [ ]   3 [ ]   4 [ ]

Comment:

5.1.2 Be appropriately visible and an active networker to reach many constituents

Unconfident   Confident
1 [ ]   2 [ ]   3 [ ]   4 [ ]

Not important in the next year   Very important in the next year
1 [ ]   2 [ ]   3 [ ]   4 [ ]

Comment:

5.1.3 Negotiate with a variety of people ground rules for shared activities

Unconfident   Confident
1 [ ]   2 [ ]   3 [ ]   4 [ ]

Not important in the next year   Very important in the next year
1 [ ]   2 [ ]   3 [ ]   4 [ ]

Comment:

5.1.4 Find ways to accommodate creative tensions

When there is tension between different ways of thinking, it is tempting for one to dominate the others. Your challenge is to turn this tension into creative collaboration. You must use what works for you: Rational argument? A picture? A phrase? A role model? Team-building exercises?

Unconfident			Confident
1 [ ]	2 [ ]	3 [ ]	4 [ ]

Not important in the next year			Very important in the next year
1 [ ]	2 [ ]	3 [ ]	4 [ ]

Comment:

5.1.5 Convert bad into good

Often something that at first sight seems bad is an opportunity to create good. Are you good at making this switch?

Unconfident			Confident
1 [ ]	2 [ ]	3 [ ]	4 [ ]

Not important in the next year			Very important in the next year
1 [ ]	2 [ ]	3 [ ]	4 [ ]

Comment:

5.1.6 Run off the ball

Exceptional footballers anticipate an opportunity from the way their team is playing and run into space to make the most of this. This only works if the other players are also skilled enough to see what is happening and to pass the ball.

Unconfident			Confident
1 [ ]	2 [ ]	3 [ ]	4 [ ]

Not important in the next year			Very important in the next year
1 [ ]	2 [ ]	3 [ ]	4 [ ]

Comment:

5.1.7 Market a message

This includes writing press releases and advertisements, and speaking in public (including radio and television)

Unconfident			Confident
1 [ ]	2 [ ]	3 [ ]	4 [ ]

Not important in the next year			Very important in the next year
1 [ ]	2 [ ]	3 [ ]	4 [ ]

Comment:

5.1.8 Use a variety of artistic expressions to communicate with others

Unconfident   Confident
1 [ ]   2 [ ]   3 [ ]   4 [ ]

Not important in the next year   Very important in the next year
1 [ ]   2 [ ]   3 [ ]   4 [ ]

Comment:

5.1.9 What other learning objectives do you have in this topic?

5.2 Retain inner peace

Experienced leaders and facilitators can often see things coming before others. They are 'visionary' and 'sensitive'. Being able to see more than others can be a lonely place, and a place full of doubt since you may have to rely on your instincts alone to get it right. Sensitivity is a double-edged sword – it allows you to see more opportunities than others, and also more threats; it helps you to feel more joy than others, and also more pain. You have to have good strategies for inner peace.

5.2.1 Use images and phrases that keep you alive in the present

Unconfident   Confident
1 [ ]   2 [ ]   3 [ ]   4 [ ]

Not important in the next year   Very important in the next year
1 [ ]   2 [ ]   3 [ ]   4 [ ]

Comment:

5.2.2 Use approaches that help you to feel balanced inside, such as mindfulness, cognitive behaviour therapy, neurolinguistic programming and meditation

Unconfident   Confident
1 [ ]   2 [ ]   3 [ ]   4 [ ]

Not important in the next year   Very important in the next year
1 [ ]   2 [ ]   3 [ ]   4 [ ]

Comment:

5.2.3 Identify and follow regular exercise routines that suit you

Unconfident   Confident
1 [ ]   2 [ ]   3 [ ]   4 [ ]

Not important in the next year   Very important in the next year
1 [ ]   2 [ ]   3 [ ]   4 [ ]

Comment:

5.2.4 Regularly interact in creative and appreciative ways with those you care about, and who care about you

Unconfident   Confident
1 [ ]   2 [ ]   3 [ ]   4 [ ]

Not important in the next year   Very important in the next year
1 [ ]   2 [ ]   3 [ ]   4 [ ]

Comment:

5.2.5 Random acts of spontaneous generosity

Unconfident   Confident
1 [ ]   2 [ ]   3 [ ]   4 [ ]

Not important in the next year   Very important in the next year
1 [ ]   2 [ ]   3 [ ]   4 [ ]

Comment:

5.2.6 What other learning objectives do you have in this topic?

5.3 Maintain a network of personal and political support

5.3.1 Create around you a 'space of sanity' – with people who are good for you and things to do that remind you of who you are and who you want to become

Have a regular schedule to revisit these things throughout the year.

Unconfident   Confident
1 [ ]   2 [ ]   3 [ ]   4 [ ]

Not important in the next year   Very important in the next year
1 [ ]   2 [ ]   3 [ ]   4 [ ]

Comment:

5.3.2 Make sufficient attendances at significant places, people and meetings to remain noticed and supported

Unconfident   Confident
1 [ ]   2 [ ]   3 [ ]   4 [ ]

Not important in the next year   Very important in the next year
1 [ ]   2 [ ]   3 [ ]   4 [ ]

Comment:

5.3.3 Nurture the stewards of organisational memory

These are people who know the history of the organisation and why this explains how it works (or not).

Unconfident   Confident
1 [ ]   2 [ ]   3 [ ]   4 [ ]

Not important in the next year   Very important in the next year
1 [ ]   2 [ ]   3 [ ]   4 [ ]

Comment:

5.3.4 Gain the trust of constituents

Do the things you said you would do, when you said you would do them; and anticipate when things need to be done.

Unconfident   Confident
1 [ ]   2 [ ]   3 [ ]   4 [ ]

Not important in the next year   Very important in the next year
1 [ ]   2 [ ]   3 [ ]   4 [ ]

Comment:

5.3.5 Nurture partners for ongoing political support

These will include those who will defend your cause in other places.

Unconfident   Confident
1 [ ]   2 [ ]   3 [ ]   4 [ ]

Not important in the next year   Very important in the next year
1 [ ]   2 [ ]   3 [ ]   4 [ ]

Comment:

5.3.6 What other learning objectives do you have in this topic?

5.4 Maintain systems to manage information

As a leader of transformational processes you have to be a 'boundary-spanner'. You will need to know details about the various organisations that you straddle, bringing an enormous amount of email traffic and basic things to update yourself about. You will need effective ways to keep up to date and systems to manage the information and audit your effectiveness.

5.4.1 Devise and maintain personal knowledge retrieval systems to obtain specific knowledge when needed

Unconfident   Confident
1 [ ]   2 [ ]   3 [ ]   4 [ ]

Not important in the next year   Very important in the next year
1 [ ]   2 [ ]   3 [ ]   4 [ ]

Comment:

5.4.2 Use a set of websites and key informants to keep you up to date

Unconfident   Confident
1 [ ]   2 [ ]   3 [ ]   4 [ ]

Not important in the next year   Very important in the next year
1 [ ]   2 [ ]   3 [ ]   4 [ ]

Comment:

5.4.3 Create networks of high-performing teams

Unconfident   Confident
1 [ ]   2 [ ]   3 [ ]   4 [ ]

Not important in the next year   Very important in the next year
1 [ ]   2 [ ]   3 [ ]   4 [ ]

Comment:

5.4.4 Lists, and lists of lists, to keep in view your commitments

Unconfident   Confident
1 [ ]   2 [ ]   3 [ ]   4 [ ]

Not important in the next year   Very important in the next year
1 [ ]   2 [ ]   3 [ ]   4 [ ]

Comment:

5.4.5 Annual timelines that remind you what you have to do and by when

Unconfident			Confident
1 [ ]	2 [ ]	3 [ ]	4 [ ]

Not important in the next year			Very important in the next year
1 [ ]	2 [ ]	3 [ ]	4 [ ]

Comment:

5.4.6 What other learning objectives do you have in this topic?

My learning plan

Having completed the questionnaire, re-read it and edit anything you now want to change. Remember, you are doing this for yourself and there are no right or wrong answers.

Then write in the table below two priority learning objectives for each of the five learning aims. if you wish, add more in the 'other priorities' from your 'wish list' in your answer sheet. You are likely to choose objectives where you scored low on confidence and high on importance. If not, ask yourself if you are making the best decision.

Write down why you have chosen the things you have chosen – this will help you later on (when things have moved on) to remind yourself why they are relevant to you at this stage.

Finally, stand back and look at all your chosen objectives to check for overall balance. Add to them any others that you think you need to learn that may not be on the curriculum.

Learning aim one: Concepts for community-oriented integrated care (COIC)

Two Priority Learning Objectives	Explain why you have chosen these objectives	Evidence
Other priorities		

Learning aim two: Evaluating COIC

Two Priority Learning Objectives	Explain why you have chosen these objectives	Evidence
Other priorities		

Learning aim three: Facilitating learning spaces

Two Priority Learning Objectives	Explain why you have chosen these objectives	Evidence
Other priorities		

Learning aim four: Orchestrating whole-system learning and change

Two Priority Learning Objectives	Explain why you have chosen these objectives	Evidence
Other priorities		

Learning aim five: Skills for personal balance

Two Priority Learning Objectives	Explain why you have chosen these objectives	Evidence
Other priorities		

Bibliography

Comprehensive primary health care

Hanlon, P., Carlisle, S., Hannah, M., Reilly D. and Lyon, A. (2011) Making the case for a 'fifth wave' in public health. *Public Health*, 125 (1): 30–36.

Macdonald, J. *Primary Health Care: medicine in its place*. London: Earthscan, 1992.

Macdonald, J. *Environments for Health: a salutogenic approach*. London: Earthscan, 2005.

NHS England. *New Care Models: supporting the design and implementation of new care models in the NHS*. 2016. www.england.nhs.uk/ourwork/new-care-models/.

WHO. *Declaration of Alma-Ata International Conference on Primary Health Care*. 6–12 September 1978. www.who.int/publications/almaata_declaration_en.pdf.

WHO. *Primary Health Care: Now More than Ever*. 2008. www.who.int/whr/2008/.

Health, identity and relationships

Antonovsky, A. *Unravelling the Mystery of Health: how people manage stress and stay well*. San Francisco, CA: Jossey-Bass, 1987.

Berne, E. *What Do You Do After You Say Hello? The psychology of human destiny*. London: Corgi, 1972.

Buber, M. (translated by Smith, R.G). *I and Thou*. London: Bloomsbury Academic, 2013 [1923].

Cherry, K. Erik Erikson's stages of psychological development. Verywell. http://psychology.about.com/od/psychosocialtheories/fl/Psychosocial-Stages-Summary-Chart.htm.

Erikson, E.H. *The Life Cycle Completed*. New York: Norton, 1998.

Leavey, C. Bird-nesting belief system. In *Why Do Women Not Attend for Cervical Smear Appointments? A participatory action research approach in Liverpool general practice* (PhD dissertation). John Moores University, 2000, pp. 252–253.

MacIntyre, A. *After Virtue: a study in moral theory*. 2nd edition. London: Duckworth, 1985.

Seedhouse, D. *Health: The foundations for achievement*. Chichester: Wiley, 1986.

Shotter, J. *Conversational Realities: constructing life through language*. London: Sage, 1993.

Stainton-Rogers, W. *Explaining Health and Illness: an exploration of diversity*. New York: Harvester Wheatsheaf, 1991.

Taylor, C. *Sources of the Self: The making of the modern identity*. Cambridge:

General practice role

Fry, J. (ed.) *Trends in General Practice*. London: RCGP, 1977.

Hart, J.T. *A New Kind of Doctor*. London: Merlin Press, 1988.

Horder, J. (2010) An account of my life. *London Journal of Primary Care*, 3: 2, 120–123. http://dx.doi.org/10.1080/17571472.2010.11493316.

Launer, J. *Narrative-based Primary Care: a practical guide.* Abingdon: Radcliffe Medical Press, 2002.

Starfield, B. *Primary Health Care: balancing health needs, services, and technology.* New York: Oxford University Press, 1998.

Toon, P.D. *A Flourishing Practice?* London: RCGP, 2014.

Tuckett, D., Boulton, M., Olson, C. and Williams, A. *Meetings Between Experts: An approach to sharing ideas in medical consultations.* London: Routledge, 1985.

Policy for integrated working

Elmore, R.F. (1979) Backward mapping: implementation research and policy decisions. *Political Science Quarterly*, 94: 601–616.

Ferlie, E. (2010) Public management 'reform' narratives and the changing organisation of primary care. *London Journal of Primary Care*, 3: 2, 76–80, DOI:10.1080/17571472.2010.11493306.

Giddens, A. *The Third Way: the renewal of social democracy.* Oxford: Polity Press in association with Blackwell Publishers Ltd, 1998.

Meads, G. *Primary Care in the Twenty-First Century: an international perspective.* Abingdon: Radcliffe, 2006.

Thomas, P., Meads, G., Moustafa, A., Nazareth, I. and Stange, K. (2008) Combined horizontal and vertical integration of care: a goal of practice-based commissioning. *Quality in Primary Care*, 16: 425–432.

Models of community-oriented integrated care

Ashton, J. and Seymour, H. *The New Public Health.* Buckingham: Open University Press, 1988.

Bromley by Bow Centre Health Partnership. www.bbbhp.co.uk.

Hart, J.T. *A New Kind of Doctor.* London: Merlin Press, 1988.

Kark, S.L. *Community-Oriented Primary Health Care.* London: Appleton-Century-Crofts, 1981.

Westfall, J.M. et al. (2014) How do rural patients benefit from the patient-centred medical home? A card study in the High Plains Research Network. *London Journal of Primary Care*, 6: 6, 136–148. DOI:10.1080/17571472.2014.11494365.

Wilson, A. *Changing Practices in Primary Care: a facilitator's handbook.* London: Health Education Authority, 1994.

Inter-organisational collaboration for community-oriented integrated care

Breton, M., Maillet, L., Haggerty, J. and Vedel, I. (2014) Mandated local health networks across the province of Québec: a better collaboration with primary care working in the communities? *London Journal of Primary Care*, 6:4, 71–78. DOI:10.1080/17571472.2014.11493420.

Bryar, R. and Bytheway, B. (eds) *Changing Primary Health Care: The Teamcare Valleys experience.* Abingdon: Blackwell Science Ltd, 1996.

Chandok, R., Unadkat, N., Nasir, L., Evans, L. and Thomas, P. (2013) How Ealing Health Networks can contribute to efficient and quality healthcare. *London Journal of Primary Care*, 5: 2, 84–86. DOI:10.1080/17571472.2013.11493385.

Evans, L., Green, S., Sharma, K., Marinho, F. and Thomas, P. (2014) Improving access to primary mental health services: are link workers the answer? *London Journal of Primary Care*, 6:2, 23–28. DOI:10.1080/17571472.2014.11493409.

Thomas, P. and Graver, L. The Liverpool intervention to promote teamwork in general practice: an action research approach. Chapter 13 in Pearson, P. and Spencer, M. (eds) *Promoting Teamwork in Primary Care: a research based approach*. London: Arnold, 1997, pp. 174–191.

Unadkat, N., Evans, L., Nasir, L., Thomas, P. and Chandok, R. (2013) Taking diabetes services out of hospital into the community. *London Journal of Primary Care*, 5: 2, 87–91. DOI:10.1 080/17571472.2013.11493386.

Leadership for integrated working

Attwood, M. et al. *Leading Change: a guide to systems working*. Bristol: Policy Press, 2003.

Thomas, P. *Integrating Primary Health Care: leading, managing facilitating*. Abingdon: Radcliffe Publishing, 2008.

Pearce, C.L. and Conger, J.A. (eds) *Shared Leadership: Reframing the Hows and Whys of Leadership*. Thousand Oaks, CA: Sage Publications, 2003.

Wheatley, M.J. *Leadership and the New Science: learning about organization from an orderly universe*. Oakland, CA:: Berrett Koehler, 1994.

Whole-system events

Bunker, B.B. and Alban, B.T. *Large Group Interventions*. San Francisco, CA: Jossey-Bass, 1997.

Harrison, O. *Open Space Technology: a user's guide*. San Francisco, CA: Berrett-Koehler, 1997.

Pratt, J., Gordon, P. and Plamping, D. *Working Whole Systems*. London: King's Fund, 1999.

Weisbord, M. and Janoff, S. *Future Search: an action guide to finding common ground in organizations and communities*. San Francisco, CA: Berrett-Koehler: 2000.

Whitney, D. and Trosten-Bloom, A. *The Power of Appreciative Inquiry*. San Francisco, CA: Berrett-Koehler, 2003.

Learning organisations and learning communities

Argyris, C. and Schon, D. *Organisational Learning II: theory, methods and practice*. Reading, MA: Addison-Wesley, 1996.

Brown, J.S. and Duguid, P. Organisational learning and communities of practice: toward a unified view of working, learning, and innovation. In Cohen, M.D. and Sproull, L.S. (eds) *Organisational Learning*. Thousand Oaks, CA: Sage, 1996, pp. 58–82.

Evans, L., Green, S., Howe, C., Sharma, K., Marinho, F., Bell, D. and Thomas, P. (2014) Improving patient and project outcomes using inter-organisational innovation, collaboration and co-design, *London Journal of Primary Care*, 6:2, 29–34 DOI:10.1080/17571472.2014.1 1493410.

Forrest, A. *Fifty Ways Towards a Learning Organisation*. Dover: The Industrial Society, 1999.

Freire, P. *Pedagogy of the Oppressed*. New York: Continuum, 2003 [1970].

Iles, V. and Sutherland, K. *Managing Change in the NHS. Organisational change: a review for health care managers, professionals and researchers*. London: London School of Hygiene and Tropical Medicine, 2001.

Kolb, D. Management and the learning process. In Starkey, K (ed.) *How Organisations Learn*. London: International Thomson Publishing, 1996, pp. 270–287.

Lewin, K. *Resolving Social Conflicts: field theory in social science. Selected papers*. Washington, DC: American Psychological Association, 1997 [originals before 1947].

McNulty, T. and Ferlie, E. *Reengineering Health Care: the complexities of organisational transformation.* Oxford: Oxford University Press, 2002.

Morgan, G. *Images of Organization.* Thousand Oaks, CA: Sage, 1997.

Senge, P. *The Fifth Discipline: the art and science of the learning organization.* London: Random House, 1999.

Social Care Institute for Excellence. *Learning Organisations: a self-assessment resources pack.* London, SCIE: 2004.

Wenger, E. *Communities of Practice: learning, meaning, and identity.* Cambridge: Cambridge University Press, 1998.

Making sense of complex co-adaptation

Boids. https://en.wikipedia.org/wiki/Boids.

Capra, F. *The Tao of Physics.* Boston: Shambhala, 1991.

Capra, F. *The Web of Life.* London: Flamingo, 1997.

Capra, F. *The Hidden Connections.* London: Flamingo, 2003.

Checkland, P. *Systems Thinking, Systems Practice.* Chichester: Wiley, 1993.

Health Foundation. *Complex Adaptive Systems.* 2010. www.health.org.uk/sites/health/files/ComplexAdaptiveSystems.pdf

Kernick, D (ed.) *Complexity and Healthcare Organization: a view from the street.* Abingdon: Radcliffe Medical Press, 2004.

Malby, B. and Fischer, M. *Tools for Change: an invitation to dance.* Chichester: Kingsham Press, 2006.

Pert, C. *Molecules of Emotion.* London: Simon & Schuster (Pocket Books), 1999.

Plesk, P. Redesigning health care with insights from the science of complex adaptive systems. In *Crossing the Quality Chasm.* Washington, DC: National Academy Press, 2001, pp. 314–317.

Stacey, R. *Complex Responsive Processes in Organizations: learning and knowledge creation.* London: Routledge, 2001.

Sweeney, K. and Griffiths, F. (eds) *Complexity and Healthcare: an introduction.* Abingdon: Radcliffe Medical Press, 2002.

Wieck, K. *Sensemaking in Organisations.* Thousand Oaks, CA: Sage, 1995.

Winston, R. and Chicot, R. (2016) The importance of early bonding on the long-term mental health and resilience of children. *London Journal of Primary Care.* http://dx.doi.org/10.1080/17571472.2015.1133012.

Research, audit and evaluation for dynamic situations

De Koning, K. and Martin, M. (eds) *Participatory Research in Health.* London: Zed Books, 1996.

Denzin, N.K. and Lincoln, Y.S. (eds) *Handbook of Qualitative Research.* Thousand Oaks, CA: Sage, 1994.

Foote-Whyte, M. *Participatory Action Research.* Newbury Park, CA: Sage, 1991.

Guba, E.G. (ed.) *The Paradigm Dialog.* Newbury Park, CA: Sage, 1990.

Guba, E.G. and Lincoln, Y.S. *Fourth Generation Evaluation.* Newbury Park, CA: Sage, 1989.

Ison, R. and Russell, D. *Agricultural Extension and Rural Development.* Cambridge: Cambridge University Press, 2000.

Janesick, V.J. The choreography of qualitative research design: minuets, improvisations, and crystallization. Chapter 13 in *Handbook of Qualitative Research.* Second edition. Thousand Oaks, CA: Sage, 2000. pp. 391–392.

Parlett, M. and Hamilton, E. Evaluation as illumination: a new approach to the study of innovatory programs. Occasional Paper. Edinburgh: Edinburgh University Centre for Research in the Educational Sciences/London: Nuffield Foundation, 1972.

Skinner, Q. (ed). *The Return of Grand Theory in the Human Sciences*. Cambridge: Cambridge University Press, 1985.

Stake, R.E. Case studies. Chapter 16 in Denzin, N.K. and Lincoln, Y.S. (eds) *Handbook of Qualitative Research*. Second Edition. Thousand Oaks, CA: Sage, 2000.

Yin, R.K. *Case Study Research*. Thousand Oaks, CA: Sage, 1994.

Evaluating complex interventions

Cordeaux, C., Hughes, A. and Elder, M. (2011) Simulating the impact of change: implementing best practice in stroke care. *London Journal of Primary Care*, 4: 1, 33–37 http://dx.doi.org/10.1080/17571472.2011.11493325.

Dhillon, A. and Godfrey, A.R. (2013) Using routinely gathered data to empower locally-led health improvements. *London Journal of Primary Care*, 5: 2, 92–95. DOI:10.1080/1757147 2.2013.11493387.

King's Fund. 2013. Experience-based co-design toolkit. https://www.kingsfund.org.uk/projects/ebcd.

Royal Society of Arts. 2015. Community capital: the value of connected communities. www.thersa.org/discover/publications-and-articles/reports/community-capital-the-value-of-connected-communities.

Stoddart, G., Gale, R., Peat, C. and McInnes, S. (2011) *Using routinely gathered data to evaluate locally led service improvements*. *London Journal of Primary Care*, 4: 1, 38–43, DOI:10.1080/17571472.2011.11493326.

Thomas, P., McDonnell, J., McCulloch, J., While, A., Bosanquet, N. and Ferlie, E. (2005) Increasing capacity for innovation in bureaucratic primary care organisations: a whole system participatory action research project. *Annals of Family Medicine*, 3: 312–317.

Integrating through networks

Health Foundation. *Leading Networks in Healthcare: learning about what works – the theory and the practice)*. London: Health Foundation, 2010.

Malby, B. and Anderson-Wallace, M. *Networks in Healthcare: managing complex relationships*. Bingley: Emerald, 2017.

Thomas, P., Graffy, J., Wallace, P. and Kirby, M. (2006) How primary care networks can help integrate academic and service initiatives in primary care. *Annals of Family Medicine*, 4: 235–239.

Non-medical approaches to health and wellbeing

Clift, S. and Camic, P. (eds) *Oxford Textbook of Creative Arts, Health, and Wellbeing: international perspectives on practice, policy and research*. Oxford: Oxford University Press, 2015.

Hallam, S. The power of music. Music Education Council. 2015. http://static1.1.sqspcdn.com/static/f/735337/25902273/1422485417967/power+of+music.pdf?token=wEczWdwUkfdyHzLbWjuPZ06g2T8%3D

Money, M. (ed.) *Health & Community: holism in practice*. Dartington: Green Books Ltd, 1993.

Royal Society for Public Health. *Arts, Health and Wellbeing Beyond the Millennium: how far have we come and where do we want to go?* London, RSPH, 2013.

Classical theories of the natural order

The Bible, Old Testament and New Testament.

Darwin, C.R. *The Origin of Species*. The Harvard Classics. New York: P.F. Collier & Son, 1909–14; Bartleby.com, 2001. www.bartleby.com/11/

Kuhn, T.S. *The Structure of Scientific Revolutions*. Chicago: University of Chicago Press, 2012.

Plato. *The Republic*. Chatham: Guild Publishing, 1990

Smith, A. *An Inquiry into the Nature and Causes of the Wealth of Nations*. London: Alex Murray & Son, 1871.

Index

Note: Page locators in *italics* refer to figures and page locators in **bold** refer to tables.